The Home Health Aide Handbook

Jetta Fuzy, RN, MS
William Leahy, MD

FOURTH EDITION

hartmanonline.com

Hartman Publishing began offering in-service education programs to long-term care facilities and home health agencies in 1994. Today we specialize in textbooks for nursing assistant and home health aide training. Students and teachers using our materials benefit from a company solely focused on educating and inspiring caregivers.

Acknowledgments

Managing Editor
Susan Alvare Hedman

Designer
Kirsten Browne

Production
Thad Castillo

Photography
Matt Pence, Pat Berrett, Art Clifton, and Dick Ruddy

Proofreaders
Kristin Calderon, Kristin Cartwright, and Joanna Owusu

Sales/Marketing
Deborah Rinker, Kendra Robertson, Erika Walker, and Belinda Midyette

Customer Service
Fran Desmond, Thomas Noble, Angela Storey, Eliza Martin, and Jeff Brown

Warehouse Coordinator
Chris Midyette

Copyright Information

Notice to Readers

Though the guidelines and procedures contained in this text are based on consultations with healthcare professionals, they should not be considered absolute recommendations. The instructor and readers should follow employer, local, state, and federal guidelines concerning healthcare practices. These guidelines change, and it is the reader's responsibility to be aware of these changes and of the policies and procedures of his or her healthcare agency.

The publisher, author, editors, and reviewers cannot accept any responsibility for errors or omissions or for any consequences from application of the information in this book and make no warranty, express or implied, with respect to the contents of the book. The publisher does not warrant or guarantee any of the products described herein or perform any analysis in connection with any of the product information contained herein.

Special Thanks

A very warm thank you goes to our insightful reviewers:

Candace S. Barth RN, BSN
Junction City, WI

Susan Meier, RN, BSN
Gloucester Township, NJ

Nelson Wood, RN, BSN, CRRN
New Hartford, NY

Gender Usage

This textbook utilizes the pronouns *he*, *his*, *she*, and *hers* interchangeably to denote care team members and clients.

Contents

VII. Caring for Yourself

VIII. Appendix

Procedure	Page

Procedures

Procedure	Page

Welcome to Hartman Publishing's Home Health Aide Handbook!

We hope you will happily place this little reference book into your purse, backpack, or your home care visit bag and leave it there so you will have it available at all times as you go about your day-to-day duties as a home health aide. This handbook will serve as a quick but comprehensive reference tool for you to use from client to client.

Features and Benefits

This book is a valuable tool for many reasons. It includes all the procedures you learned in your home health aide training program, plus references to abbreviations, medical terms, care guidelines for specific diseases, and an appendix where you can write down important names and phone numbers. For certified nursing assistants moving to home care, we have included information on making the transition from facilities to homes. In addition, this book contains all of the federal requirements for home health aides, so it can also be used in a basic training program.

We have divided the book into eight parts and assigned each part its own colored tab, which you will see at the top of every page.

I. Defining Home Health Services

II. Foundation of Client Care

III. Understanding Clients

IV. Client Care

V. Special Clients, Special Needs

VI. Home Management and Nutrition

VII. Caring for Yourself

VIII. Appendix

You will find **key terms** throughout the text. Explanations for these terms are in the Glossary section of the Appendix of this book. Common Disorders, Guidelines, and Observing and Reporting are also colored for easy reference. Procedures are indicated with a black bar. There is also an index in the back of the book. We will be updating this guide periodically, so don't hesitate to let us know what you would like to see in the next handbook we publish. Contact us at

Hartman Publishing, Inc.
1313 Iron Avenue SW
Albuquerque, NM 87102
Phone: (505) 291-1274
Fax: (505) 291-1284
Web: hartmanonline.com
E-mail: orders@hartmanonline.com
Twitter: @HartmanPub

Beginning and ending steps in care procedures

For most care procedures, these steps should be performed. Understanding why they are important will help you remember to perform each step every time care is provided.

Beginning Steps

Wash your hands.

Handwashing provides for infection prevention. Nothing fights infection like performing consistent, proper hand hygiene. Handwashing may need to be done more than once during a procedure. Practice Standard Precautions with every client.

Explain the procedure to client, speaking clearly, slowly, and directly. Maintain face-to-face contact whenever possible.

Clients have a right to know exactly what care you will provide. It promotes understanding, cooperation, and independence. Clients are able to do more for themselves if they know what needs to happen.

Provide privacy for the client.

Doing this maintains the client's right to privacy and dignity. Providing for privacy is not simply a courtesy; it is a legal right.

If the bed is adjustable, adjust bed to a safe level, usually waist high. If the bed is movable, lock bed wheels.

If the client has an adjustable bed, locking the bed wheels is an important safety measure. It ensures that the bed will not move as you are performing care. Raising the bed helps you to remember to use proper body mechanics. This prevents injury to you and to the client.

Ending Steps

Return bed to lowest position.	Lowering an adjustable bed provides for the client's safety.
Wash your hands.	Handwashing is the most important thing you can do to prevent the spread of infection.
Document the procedure and your observations.	You will often be the person who spends the most time with a client, so you are in the best position to note any changes in a client's condition. Every time you provide care, observe the client's physical and mental capabilities, as well as the condition of his or her body. For example, a change in a client's ability to dress himself may signal a greater problem. After you have finished giving care, document the care properly. Do not record care before it is given. If you do not document the care you gave, legally it did not happen.

In addition to the beginning and ending steps listed above, remember to follow infection prevention guidelines. Even if a procedure in this book does not tell you to wear gloves or other PPE, there may be times when it is appropriate.

I. Defining Home Health Services

Home Health Care

Home health aides (HHAs) provide assistance to the chronically ill, the elderly, and family caregivers who need relief from the stress of caregiving. Many home health aides also work in assisted living facilities, which provide independent living in a homelike group environment, with professional care available as needed. As advances in medicine and technology extend the lives of people with **chronic** illnesses, the number of people needing health care will increase. The need for home health aides will also increase.

Payers

Agencies pay HHAs from payments they receive from these payers:

- Insurance companies
- Government programs like **Medicare** and **Medicaid**
- **Health maintenance organizations** (**HMOs**)
- **Preferred provider organizations** (**PPOs**)
- Individual clients or family members

The Centers for Medicare & Medicaid Services (CMS) is a federal agency within the U.S. Department of Health and Human Services. CMS runs the Medicare and Medicaid programs at the federal level.

Medicare pays agencies a fixed fee for a 60-day period of care based on a client's condition. If the cost of providing care exceeds the payment, the agency loses money. If the care provided costs less than the payment, the agency makes money. For these reasons, home health agencies must pay close attention to costs. Because all payers monitor the quality of care provided, the way in which work is documented is very important. CMS' payment system for home care is called the *home health prospective payment system* or *HH PPS*.

Purpose of Home Care

One of the most important reasons for offering health care in the home is that most people who are ill or disabled feel more comfortable at home. Health care in familiar surroundings improves mental and physical well-being. It has proven to be a major factor in the healing process.

Agency Structure

Clients who need home care are referred to a home health agency by their doctors. They can also be referred by a hospital discharge planner, a social services agency, the state or local department of public health, the welfare office, a local Agency on Aging, or a senior center. Clients and family members may also choose an agency that meets their needs. Once an agency is chosen and the doctor has made a referral, a staff member performs an assessment of the client. This determines how the care needs can best be met. The home environment will also be evaluated to determine whether it is safe for the client.

Home health agencies employ many home health aides (HHAs) and certified nursing assistants (CNAs or NAs). The services provided depend on the size of the agency. Small agencies may provide basic nursing care, personal care, and housekeeping services. Larger agencies may provide speech, physical, and occupational therapies and medical social work. Common services provided include medical-surgical nursing care, including medication management, wound care, care of different types of tubes, and care for different diseases. Services also include intravenous infusion therapy; maternal, pediatric, and newborn nursing care; nutrition therapy; medical social work; personal care; medical equipment rental and service; pharmacy services; and hospice services. All home health agencies have professional staff who make decisions about what services are needed (Fig. 1-1).

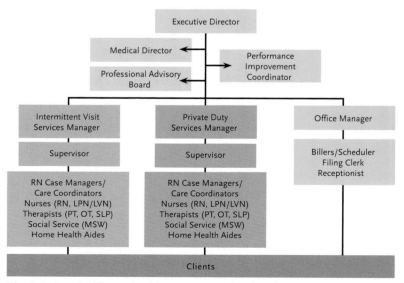

Fig. 1-1. *A typical home health agency organization chart.*

HHA's Role

An HHA may be assigned to spend a certain number of hours each day or week with a client to provide care and services. While the client care plan and assignments are developed by the supervisor or case manager, input from all members of the care team is needed. All HHAs are under the supervision of a skilled, licensed professional: a nurse, a physical therapist, a speech-language pathologist, or an occupational therapist.

Working in Clients' Homes

In some ways, working as a home health aide is similar to working as a nursing assistant. Most of the basic medical procedures and many of the personal care procedures will be the same. However, some aspects of working in the home are different:

- **Housekeeping**: An HHA may have housekeeping responsibilities, including cooking, cleaning, laundry, and grocery shopping, for at least some clients.
- **Family contact**: An HHA may have a lot more contact with clients' family members in the home than she would in a facility.
- **Independence**: An HHA will work independently. A supervisor will monitor her work, but the HHA will spend most hours working with clients without direct supervision. Thus, the HHA must be a responsible and independent worker.
- **Communication**: Communication skills are important. An HHA must keep herself informed of changes in the client care plan. She must also keep others informed of changes she observes in the client and the client's environment.
- **Transportation**: An HHA will have to get herself from one client's home to another. She will need to have a dependable car or be able to use public transportation. An HHA may also face bad weather conditions. Clients need care—rain, snow, or sleet.
- **Safety**: An HHA needs to be aware of personal safety when traveling alone to visit clients. She should be aware of her surroundings, walk confidently, and avoid dangerous situations.
- **Flexibility**: Each client's home will be different. An HHA will need to adapt to the changes in environment.
- **Working environment**: In home care, the layout of rooms, stairs, lack of equipment, cramped bathrooms, rugs, clutter, and even pets can complicate caregiving.
- **Client's home**: In a client's home, an HHA is a guest. She needs to be respectful of the client's property and customs.

- **Client's comfort**: One of the best things about home care is that it allows clients to stay in the familiar and comfortable surroundings of their own homes. This can help most clients recover or adapt to their condition more quickly.

An HHA is part of a team of health professionals that includes doctors, nurses, social workers, therapists, and specialists. The client and client's family are considered a very important part of the team. Everyone involved will work closely together to help clients recover from illnesses or injuries. If full recovery is not possible, the team will help clients do as much as they can for themselves.

The Care Team

Clients will have different needs and problems. Healthcare professionals with different kinds of education and experience will help care for them. This group is known as the *care team*. Members of the healthcare team include the following:

Home Health Aide (HHA): The home health aide performs assigned tasks, such as taking vital signs. The HHA also provides routine personal care, such as bathing clients or preparing meals. Daily personal care tasks such as bathing; caring for skin, nails, hair, and teeth; dressing; toileting; eating and drinking; walking; and transferring are referred to as **activities of daily living** (**ADLs**). Assisting with ADLs is a major part of the HHA's responsibilities. HHAs spend more time with clients than other care team members. They act as the "eyes and ears" of the team. Observing and reporting changes in a client's condition or abilities is a very important duty of the HHA.

Case Manager or Supervisor: Usually a registered nurse, a case manager or a supervisor is assigned to each client by the home health agency. The case manager, with input from other team members, creates the basic care plan for the client. He or she monitors any changes that are observed and reported by the HHA. The case manager also makes changes in the client care plan when necessary.

Registered Nurse (RN): In a home health agency, a registered nurse coordinates, manages, and provides care. RNs also supervise and train HHAs. They develop the HHA's assignments.

Doctor (MD or DO): A doctor's job is to diagnose disease or disability and prescribe treatment. A doctor generally decides when patients need home health care and can refer them to home health agencies.

Physical Therapist (PT or DPT): A physical therapist evaluates a person and develops a treatment plan. Goals are to increase movement, improve circulation, promote healing, reduce pain, prevent disability, and regain or maintain mobility. A PT gives therapy in the form of heat, cold, massage, ultrasound, electrical stimulation, and exercise to muscles, bones, and joints.

Occupational Therapist (OT): An occupational therapist helps clients learn to adapt to disabilities. An OT may help train clients to perform activities of daily living (ADLs) such as dressing, eating, and bathing.

Speech-Language Pathologist (SLP): A speech-language pathologist, or speech therapist, identifies communication disorders, addresses factors involved in recovery, and develops a plan of care to meet recovery goals. An SLP teaches exercises to help the client improve or overcome speech problems. An SLP also evaluates a person's ability to swallow food and drink.

Registered Dietitian (RDT): A registered dietitian teaches clients and their families about special diets to improve their health and help them manage their illness. RDTs may supervise the preparation and service of food and educate others about healthy nutritional habits.

Medical Social Worker (MSW): A medical social worker determines clients' needs and helps them get support services, such as counseling, meal services, and financial assistance.

Client and Client's Family: The client is an important member of the care team. The client has the right to make decisions and choices about his or her own care. The client's family may also be involved in these decisions. The family is a great source of information. They know the client's personal preferences, history, diet, rituals, and routines. They may also be learning about the care provided, as they may care for the client when home health care ends. The care team revolves around the client and his or her condition, treatment, and progress. Without the client, there is no care team.

The Care Plan

The client care plan is individualized for each client. It is developed to help achieve the goals of care. It lists tasks that the care team, including home health aides, must perform. It states how often these tasks should be done and how they should be carried out.

The care plan is a guide to help the client be as healthy as possible. **Activities not listed on the care plan should not be performed**. The HHA care plan is part of the overall plan of care. It must be followed very carefully.

Care planning should involve input from the client and/or the family, as well as health professionals. Professionals will assess the client's physical, financial, social, and psychological needs. After the doctor prescribes treatment, the supervisor, nurses, and other care team members create the care plan. Many factors are considered when creating the care plan. They include the client's health and physical condition, diagnosis, treatment, goals or expectations, any additional services needed, and the client's home environment and family.

Multiple care plans may be necessary for some clients. In these situations, the supervisor will coordinate the client's overall care. There will be one care plan for the HHA to follow. There will be separate care plans for other providers, such as the physical therapist.

Care plans must be updated as the client's condition changes. Reporting changes and problems to the supervisor is a very important duty of the home health aide. That is how the care team revises care plans to meet the client's changing needs (Fig. 1-2).

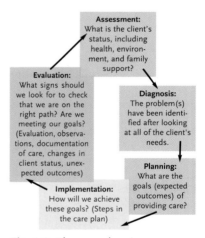

Fig. 1-2. *The care planning process.*

Chain of Command

A home health aide carries out instructions given by a nurse. The nurse is acting on the instructions of a doctor or other member of the care team. This **chain of command** describes the line of authority and helps to make sure that clients get proper health care. It also protects employees and employers from liability. **Liability** is a legal term that means someone can be held responsible for harming someone else. For example, imagine that something an HHA does for a client harms that client. However, what the HHA did was in the care plan and was done according to policy and procedure. In that case, he may not be liable, or responsible, for hurting the client. However, if an HHA does something not in the care plan that harms a client, he could be held responsible. That is why it is important for the team to follow instructions in the care plan and for the agency to have a chain of command (Fig. 1-3).

Every state grants the right to practice various jobs in health care through licensure. Examples include a license to practice nursing, medicine, or physical therapy. Each member of the care team works within his or her scope of practice. A **scope of practice** defines the tasks that healthcare providers are allowed to do and how to do them correctly.

Home health aides must understand what they can and cannot do. This is important so that they do not harm clients or involve themselves or their employer in a lawsuit. Some states certify that a home health aide is qualified to work. However, home health aides are not licensed healthcare providers. Everything they do in their job is assigned by a licensed healthcare professional. They work under the authority of another person's license. That is why these professionals will show great interest in what HHAs do and how they do it.

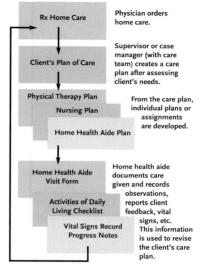

Fig. 1-3. *The chain of command describes the line of authority and helps ensure that the client receives proper care.*

Policies and Procedures

All agencies have manuals outlining their policies and procedures. A **policy** is a course of action that should be taken every time a certain situation occurs. For example, a very basic policy is that healthcare information must remain confidential. A **procedure** is a particular method, or way, of doing something. For example, an agency will have a procedure for reporting information about clients. The procedure explains what form to complete, when and how often to fill it out, and to whom it is given.

Common policies and procedures at home health agencies include the following:

- All client information must remain confidential.
- The client's care plan must always be followed. Tasks not listed in the care plan or approved by the supervisor should not be done.

- HHAs must report to the supervisor at regular arranged times, and more often if necessary.
- HHAs must report important events or changes in clients to their supervisor.
- Personal problems must not be discussed with the client or the client's family.
- HHAs must be punctual and dependable.
- Deadlines for documentation and paperwork must be met.
- HHAs must provide all client care in a pleasant, professional manner.
- HHAs must not give or accept gifts.

Employers will have policies and procedures for every client care situation. Procedures may seem long and complicated, but each step is important.

Professionalism

Professional means having to do with work or a job. The opposite of professional is *personal*. Personal refers to life outside a job, such as family, friends, and home life. Professionalism is about behaving properly when on the job. It includes dressing appropriately and speaking well. It also includes being on time, finishing assignments, and reporting to the supervisor. For an HHA, professionalism means following the care plan, making important observations, and reporting accurately.

Following policies and procedures is an important part of professionalism. Clients, coworkers, and supervisors respect employees who behave in a professional way. Professionalism helps people keep their jobs. It may also help them earn promotions and raises.

A professional relationship with clients includes the following:

- Keeping a positive attitude
- Arriving on time, doing tasks efficiently, and leaving on time
- Finishing an assignment
- Doing only the tasks assigned
- Keeping all clients' information confidential
- Being polite and cheerful at all times (Fig. 1-4)

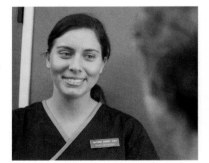

Fig. 1-4. HHAs are expected to be polite and cheerful in all circumstances.

- Not discussing personal problems
- Not making personal phone calls or sending or reading texts or emails when working
- Not using profanity, even if a client does
- Listening to the client
- Never giving or accepting gifts
- Calling the client *Mr.*, *Mrs.*, *Ms.*, or *Miss*, and his or her last name, or using the name he or she prefers
- Always explaining care before providing it
- Following practices, such as handwashing, to protect care providers and clients

A professional relationship with employers includes the following:

- Completing assignments efficiently
- Always following policies and procedures
- Documenting and reporting carefully and correctly
- Reporting problems with clients or assignments
- Reporting anything that keeps an HHA from completing assignments
- Asking questions when the HHA does not know or understand something
- Taking directions or criticism without getting upset
- Being cleanly and neatly dressed and groomed, following all agency policies (Fig. 1-5)
- Always being on time
- Telling the employer if the HHA cannot report to work
- Following the chain of command
- Participating in education programs
- Being a positive role model for the agency

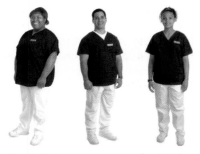

Fig. 1-5. *Proper grooming for HHAs includes wearing a uniform that has been washed and ironed. Hair should be clean and brushed, and long hair should be tied back. Shoes should be clean and comfortable.*

Home health aides must be **compassionate**, **empathetic**, sympathetic, and honest. They must also be **tactful**, **conscientious**, dependable, patient, respectful, unprejudiced, and tolerant.

Legal and Ethical Aspects

Ethics and laws guide behavior. **Ethics** are the knowledge of right and wrong. An ethical person has a sense of duty toward others. He tries to do what is right. **Laws** are rules set by the government to help people live peacefully together and to ensure order and safety.

Ethics and laws are very important in health care. They protect people receiving care and guide those giving care. Home health aides and all care team members should be guided by a code of ethics. They must know the laws that apply to their jobs.

Guidelines: Legal and Ethical Behavior

G   Be honest at all times.

G   Protect clients' privacy and confidentiality.

G   Report abuse or suspected abuse of clients. Assist clients in report-ing abuse if they wish to make a complaint of abuse.

G   Follow the care plan and assignments.

G   Do not perform any unassigned tasks or tasks outside your scope of practice.

G   Report all client observations and incidents to the supervisor.

G   Document accurately and promptly.

G   Follow rules on safety and infection prevention, including the Occupational Safety and Health Administration (OSHA) rules about bloodborne pathogens, Standard Precautions, and tuberculosis.

G   Do not accept gifts or tips.

G   Do not become personally or sexually involved with clients or their family members or friends.

G   Do not bring friends or family members with you to clients' homes.

Maintaining Boundaries

In professional relationships, boundaries must be set. Boundaries are the limits to or within relationships. Home health aides, like other professionals, are guided by ethics and laws which set limits for their relationships with clients. These boundaries help support a healthy client-worker relationship. Working in clients' homes may make it more difficult to honor the boundaries of professional rela-tionships. Clients may feel that HHAs are their friends because they are in their homes. If an HHA and a client become personally involved with each other, it becomes more difficult to enforce rules.

For instance, an HHA may want to give a client extra help or let her skip exercise she dislikes. The client may expect the HHA to break the rules because she thinks they are friends. Emotional attachments to clients are unprofessional and may weaken an HHA's judgment. HHAs should be friendly, warm, and caring with clients, but they should behave professionally and stay within the limits of set boundaries. Agency rules and the care plan's instructions should be followed. They are in place for everyone's protection.

Advance Directives

Advance directives are legal documents that allow people to choose what medical care they wish to have if they are unable to make those decisions themselves. Advance directives can also name someone to make decisions for a person if that person becomes ill or disabled. Living wills, durable powers of attorney for health care, and health care proxies are examples of advance directives. By law, advance directives must be honored. HHAs should respect each client's decisions about advance directives. This is a very personal and private matter. HHAs should not make comments about clients' choices to anyone.

Clients' rights relate to how clients must be treated. They provide an ethical code of conduct for healthcare workers. Home health agencies give clients a list of these rights and review each right with them. Many states require home health agencies to provide their clients with abuse hotline numbers. By law, HHAs must report suspected cases of abuse.

Client's Bill of Rights

Home health clients and their formal caregivers have a right to not be discriminated against on the basis of race, color, religion, national origin, age, sex, gender, sexual orientation, or disability. Furthermore, clients and caregivers have a right to mutual respect and dignity, including respect for property. Caregivers are prohibited from accepting personal gifts and borrowing from clients.

Clients have the right

- To have relationships with home health providers that are based on honesty and ethical standards of conduct;
- To be informed of the procedure they can follow to lodge complaints with the home health provider about the care that is, or fails to be, furnished and about a lack of respect for property;

- To know about the disposition of such complaints;
- To voice their grievances without fear of discrimination or reprisal for having done so; and
- To be advised of the telephone number and hours of operation of the state's home care hotline which receives questions and complaints about local home care agencies, including complaints about implementation of advance directive requirements.

Clients have the right

- To be notified in advance about the care that is to be furnished, the disciplines of the caregivers who will furnish the care, and the frequency of the proposed visits;
- To be advised of any change in the plan of care before the change is made;
- To participate in planning care and planning changes in care, and to be advised that they have the right to do so;
- To be informed in writing of rights under state law to make decisions concerning medical care, including the right to accept or refuse treatment and the right to formulate advance directives;
- To be notified of the expected outcomes of care and any obstacles or barriers to treatment;*
- To be informed in writing of policies and procedures for implementing advance directives, including any limitations if the provider cannot implement an advance directive on the basis of conscience;

- To have healthcare providers comply with advance directives in accordance with state law;
- To receive care without condition or discrimination based on the execution of advance directives; and
- To refuse services without fear of reprisal or discrimination.

* The home care provider or the client's physician may be forced to refer the client to another source of care if the client's refusal to comply with the plan of care threatens to compromise the provider's commitment to quality care.

Clients have the right

- To confidentiality of the medical record, as well as information about their health, social, and financial circumstances and about what takes place in the home; and
- To expect the home care provider to release information only as required by law or authorized by the client and to be informed of procedures for disclosure.

Clients have the right

- To be informed of the extent to which payment may be expected from Medicare, Medicaid, or any other payer known to the home care provider;
- To be informed of the charges that will not be covered by Medicare;
- To be informed of the charges for which the client may be liable;
- To receive this information orally and in writing before care is initiated and within 30 calen-

dar days of the date the home care provider becomes aware of any changes; and

- To have access, upon request, to all bills for service the client has received, regardless of whether the bills are paid out-of-pocket or by another party.

Clients have the right

- To receive care of the highest quality;
- In general, to be admitted by a home health provider only if it has the resources needed to provide the care safely and at the required level of intensity, as determined by a professional assessment; a provider with less than optimal resources may nevertheless admit the client if a more appropriate provider is not available, but only after fully informing the client of the provider's limitations and the lack of suitable alternative arrangements; and
- To be told what to do in the case of an emergency.

The home health provider shall assure that

- All medically-related home care is provided in accordance with physicians' orders and that a plan of care specifies the services and their frequency and duration; and
- All medically-related personal care is provided by an appro-

priately trained home health aide who is supervised by a nurse or other qualified home care professional.

Clients have the responsibility

- To notify the provider of changes in their condition (e.g., hospitalization, changes in the plan of care, symptoms to be reported);
- To follow the plan of care;
- To notify the provider if the visit schedule needs to be changed;
- To inform providers of the existence of any changes made to advance directives;
- To advise the provider of any problems or dissatisfaction with the services provided;
- To provide a safe environment for care to be provided; and
- To carry out mutually-agreed-upon responsibilities.

To satisfy the Medicare certification requirements, the Centers for Medicare & Medicaid Services (CMS) requires that agencies

1. Give a copy of the Bill of Rights to each client during the admission process.
2. Explain the Bill of Rights to the client and document that this has been done.

Agencies may have clients sign a copy of the Client's Bill of Rights to acknowledge receipt.

Guidelines: Protecting Clients' Rights

G   Never **abuse** a client **physically**, **psychologically**, **verbally**, or **sexually**.

G   Watch for and report to your supervisor any signs of abuse or **neglect**.

G Call the client by the name he or she prefers.

G Involve clients in planning. Allow them to make as many choices as possible about when, where, and how care is performed.

G Always explain a procedure to the client before performing it.

G Provide for privacy before giving care. Do not unnecessarily expose a client during care.

G Respect a client's refusal of care. Report the refusal to your supervisor immediately.

G Tell your supervisor if a client has questions about the goals of care or the care plan.

G Be truthful when documenting care.

G Do not talk or gossip about a client.

G Knock and ask permission before entering a client's room.

G Do not open a client's mail or look through his belongings.

G Do not accept gifts or money from a client.

G Report any questionable financial practices to your supervisor.

G Respect clients' property. Handle personal possessions carefully.

G Report observations regarding a client's condition or care.

Observing and Reporting: Abuse and Neglect

O/R Physical abuse—unexplained injuries including burns, bruises, and bone injuries

O/R Psychological abuse—complaints of anxiety, signs of stress, withdrawal from others, or fear of family members, friends, or authority figures

O/R Neglect (**active** or **passive**)—signs of lack of care, such as incontinence briefs not changed, soiled bedding, pressure ulcers, or lack of food in the house

Negligence means actions, or the failure to act or provide the proper care for a client, resulting in unintended injury. Some examples of negligence include the following:

• An HHA does not notice that a client's dentures do not fit properly. The client does not eat enough and becomes malnourished.

• An HHA does not observe that a client's eyesight is getting worse. Corrective measures are not taken, and the client falls and is injured.

• An HHA forgets to lock a client's wheelchair before transferring her. The client falls and is injured.

- An HHA fails to provide care for the client as assigned in the care plan.

To respect **confidentiality** means to keep private things private. HHAs will learn confidential (private) information about clients. They may learn about a client's health, finances, and relationships. Ethically and legally, they must protect this information. HHAs should not share information about clients with anyone other than the care team.

Congress passed the **Health Insurance Portability and Accountability Act** (**HIPAA**) (hhs.gov/ocr/privacy) in 1996. It has been further defined and revised since then. Congress passed this law to help keep health information private and secure. All healthcare organizations must take special steps to protect health information. Their employees can be fined and/or imprisoned if they do not follow special rules to protect privacy.

Under HIPAA, a person's protected health information (PHI) must be kept private. Examples of PHI include name, address, telephone number, social security number, email address, and medical record number. Only those who must have information to provide care or to process records should know this information. They must protect the information so it does not become known or used by anyone else. It must be kept confidential.

HIPAA applies to all healthcare providers, including doctors, nurses, home health aides, and any other care team members. HHAs cannot give any information about a client to anyone who is not directly involved in the client's care unless the client gives official consent or unless the law requires it. For example, if a neighbor asks an HHA how a client is doing, she should reply, "I'm sorry but I cannot share that information. It's confidential." That is the correct response to anyone who does not have a legal reason to know about the client.

All healthcare workers must follow HIPAA regulations, no matter where they are or what they are doing. There are serious penalties for violating these rules, including fines and prison sentences.

Maintaining confidentiality is a legal and ethical obligation. It is part of respecting clients and their rights. Discussing a client's care or personal affairs with anyone other than members of the care team violates the law.

II. Foundation of Client Care

Communication

Communication is the process of exchanging information with others. It is a process of sending and receiving messages. People communicate with signs and symbols, such as words, drawings, and pictures. They also communicate through their behavior.

Effective communication is a critical part of a home health aide's job. HHAs must communicate with supervisors, the care team, clients, and family members. A client's health depends on how well HHAs communicate observations and concerns to the supervisor. They must also be able to communicate clearly and respectfully in stressful or confusing situations.

Clients may display **combative**, meaning violent or hostile, behavior. Such behavior may include hitting, pushing, kicking, or verbal attacks. It may be the result of an illness or disease. It may also be due to frustration. Or it may just be part of someone's personality. In general, combative behavior is not a reaction to a caregiver. It should not be taken personally. HHAs should always report and document combative behavior. Even if they are not upset by the behavior, the care team needs to be aware of it.

Guidelines: Combative Behavior

G   Block physical blows or step out of the way, but never hit back.

G   Allow the client time to calm down before the next interaction.

G   Ensure the client is safe and give him or her space.

G   Remain calm. Lower the tone of your voice.

G   Be flexible and patient.

G   Stay neutral. Do not respond to verbal attacks. Do not argue or accuse the client of wrongdoing.

G   Do not use gestures that could frighten or startle the client.

G   Be reassuring and supportive.

G   Consider what provoked the client.

G   Report inappropriate behavior to your supervisor.

Barriers to Communication

Communication can be blocked or disrupted in many ways. The following are some barriers and ways for HHAs to avoid them:

- **Client does not hear HHA, does not hear correctly, or does not understand.** Face the client. Speak slowly and clearly. Do not shout, whisper, or mumble. Speak in a low voice, using a pleasant tone.

- **Client is difficult to understand.** Be patient and take time to listen. Ask client to repeat or explain the message. State the message in your own words to make sure you have understood.

- **HHA, client, or others use words that are not understood.** Do not use medical terminology with clients or their families. Use simple, everyday words. Ask what a word means if you are not sure.

- **HHA uses slang or profanity.** Avoid using slang words. They are unprofessional and may not be understood. Do not use profanity, even if the client does.

- **HHA uses clichés.** Clichés are phrases that are used over and over again and do not really mean anything. For example, "Everything will be fine" is a cliché. Instead of using a cliché, listen to what a client is really saying. Respond with a meaningful message.

- **HHA responds with "Why?"** Avoid asking "Why?" when a client makes a statement. "Why" questions can make people feel defensive.

- **HHA gives advice.** Do not offer your opinion or give medical advice. Giving medical advice is not within an HHA's scope of practice.

- **Client speaks a different language.** Speak slowly and clearly. Keep your messages short and simple. You may need to use pictures or gestures to communicate.

- **HHA or client uses nonverbal communication. Nonverbal communication** can change a message. Be aware of your body language and gestures. Look for nonverbal messages from clients and clarify them.

Oral Reports

HHAs must be able to make brief, accurate oral and written reports to clients and staff. Careful observations are used to make these reports and are important to the health and well-being of all clients. Signs and symptoms that should be reported will be discussed throughout this book. Some observations will need to be reported immediately to the supervisor. Anything that endangers clients should be reported immediately, including the following:

- Falls

- Chest pain
- Severe headache
- Difficulty breathing
- Abnormal pulse, respirations, or blood pressure
- Change in mental status
- Sudden weakness or loss of mobility
- High fever
- Loss of consciousness
- Change in level of consciousness
- Bleeding
- Change in client's condition
- Bruises, abrasions, or other signs of possible abuse

When clients report symptoms, events, or feelings, the HHA should have them repeat what they have said and ask for more information. The HHA should ask open-ended questions that need more than a "yes" or "no" answer. For example, asking the client, "Did you sleep well last night?" could easily be answered "yes" or "no." However, asking the client, "Tell me about your night and how you slept," is more likely to encourage the client to offer facts and details.

Oral reports may also be used to tell the team about an HHA's experiences with a client or family member, or to share observations of the client's condition and care. When making the report, facts, not opinions, are most useful to the care team. Two kinds of factual information are needed in reporting. Objective information is based on what a person sees, hears, touches, or smells. Objective information is collected by using the senses. Subjective information is something a person cannot or did not observe. It is based on something that the client reported that may or may not be true. The nurse or doctor needs factual information in order to make decisions about care and treatment. However, both objective and subjective reports are valuable.

For oral reports, the HHA should write notes so that important details are not forgotten. Following an oral report, the HHA must document when, why, about what, and to whom an oral report was given.

Sometimes a supervisor or another member of the care team will give an HHA a brief oral report on a client. The HHA should listen carefully and take notes if needed. She should ask about anything she does not understand. At the end of the report, the HHA can restate what she has been told to make sure she understands.

Using the Senses

In order to report accurately, HHAs must observe clients, their families, and their homes. To observe accurately, HHAs need to use as many senses as possible to gather information.

- **Sight**. The HHA should look for changes in the client's appearance. These include rashes, redness, paleness, swelling, discharge, weakness, sunken eyes, and changes in posture or gait (walking). Changes in the home should be observed. Does the home appear disorganized or dirty? Is food needed? Are there any safety hazards?

- **Hearing.** The HHA should listen to what the client says about his condition, family, or needs. Is the client speaking clearly and making sense? Does he show emotions such as anger, frustration, or sadness? Is his breathing normal? Does he wheeze, gasp, or cough? Is the area quiet enough for him to rest as needed?

- **Touch.** Does the client's skin feel hot or cool, moist or dry? Is his pulse rate regular? The HHA should use her sense of touch to test the bath water and the home's heating or cooling system.

- **Smell**. Are there any odors coming from the client's body? Odors could indicate poor bathing, infections, or **incontinence**. Breath odor could suggest use of alcohol or tobacco, indigestion, or poor mouth care. Odors in the home may suggest that housecleaning or repairs are needed. Food odors could indicate spoilage.

Documentation

Maintaining current documentation means keeping a record of everything an HHA does and observes during a client visit. Careful documentation is important for these reasons:

- It is the only way to guarantee clear and complete communication between all the members of the care team.

- Documentation is a legal record of every part of a client's treatment. It is proof that a visit was actually made. Medical charts can be used in court as legal evidence.

- Documentation helps protect HHAs and their employers from liability by proving what they did while caring for clients.

- Documentation gives an up-to-date record of the status and care of each client.

Visit records, progress notes, or clinical notes are the notes an HHA makes each time she visits a client. These notes serve as a record of the visit and the care provided. Visit records also document observations of the client's condition, change, or progress (improvement).

Guidelines: Careful Documentation

G   Document care immediately after the visit. This makes important details easier to remember. **Do not record care before it has been given.**

G   Think about what you want to say before documenting. Be brief and clear.

G   Use facts, not opinions. For example, "Client has lost 2 lbs. Did not finish lunch," reports facts. It is more useful than, "Client is thin and won't eat." When reporting something a client or family member told you, put the words in quotation marks (" "). Document the tasks that you performed, assisted with, or observed.

G   Use black ink when documenting by hand. Write neatly.

G   If you make a mistake, draw one line through it. Write the correct information. Put your initials and the date. Do not erase something you have written. Do not use correction fluid.

G   Sign your full name and title (for example, Steven Weitzman, HHA). Write the date after each day's visit notes.

G   Document as specified in the care plan. Some agencies have a check-off sheet for documenting care. It may be called an *ADL* (activities of daily living) or *flow sheet.*

An incident is an accident, problem, or unexpected event during the course of care. It is something that is not part of the normal routine. **Incident reports** must be completed when an incident occurs during a visit. Incident reports should be done when any of the following occurs:

• A client falls (all falls must be reported, even if the client says he or she is fine)

• An HHA or a client breaks or damages something

• An HHA makes a mistake in care

• A client or a family member makes a request that is out of the HHA's scope of practice or is not on the assignment sheet

• A client or a family member makes sexual advances or remarks

• Anything happens that makes an HHA feel uncomfortable, threatened, or unsafe

- An HHA gets injured on the job
- An HHA is exposed to blood or body fluids

Reporting and documenting incidents is done to protect everyone involved. This includes the client, the employer, and the home health aide. HHAs must report any incident, including job-related injuries, as soon as possible. An incident must be reported before leaving the client's home. The HHA should always check with her supervisor before completing the report. Every home health agency has its own policies and procedures for incident reporting.

Telephone Communication

An HHA may use the telephone to communicate with a supervisor. He should always ask permission before using a client's phone. An HHA may also need to answer the phone for clients and take messages.

Guidelines: Telephone Communication

When making a call, follow these steps:

G   Always identify yourself before asking to speak to someone. Never ask, "Who is this?" when someone answers your call.

G   After you have identified yourself, ask for the person with whom you need to speak.

G   If the person you are calling is available, identify yourself again. State why you are calling.

G   If the person is not available, ask if you can leave a message. Always leave a message, even if it is only to say you called. The message shows that you were trying to reach someone.

G   Leave a brief and clear message. Do not give more information than necessary.

G   Thank the person who takes the message for you. Always be polite over the telephone, as you would be in person.

When answering a call, follow these steps:

G   Always identify yourself and your position first.

G   Do not ask for more information than the client needs to return the call: a name and phone number is enough.

G   Do not give out any information about your client. Simply say, "Mr. Schmidt is not available right now. May I take a message?" Write down the name and number of the caller. Tell the client about the call.

Infection Prevention

This section provides a brief review of concepts and skills regarding infection prevention, Standard Precautions, and Transmission-Based Precautions.

Preventing the spread of infection is as important in the home as in any other healthcare setting. The difference is that in the home, a great responsibility rests on the caregiver. In a facility, proper equipment is provided, and policies and procedures are enforced. HHAs should be familiar with their agency's **infection prevention** practices. These include all policies and procedures affecting day-to-day tasks. There are no high faucets or deep sinks with special liquid soap and paper towel dispensers in most homes. HHAs will be expected to adapt to what is actually available to use. Therefore, the HHA should assess the home for available resources first. He can plan how he will follow the appropriate standards of care. This includes the proper precautions to prevent and control infection.

Home Care Bag

In some situations, it may be a good idea for the HHA to carry a home care bag. This bag can contain needed supplies, such as gloves, special handwashing wipes or soaps, paper towels, alcohol wipes, and a personal protective equipment (PPE) kit for emergencies. This special bag, which could be something like a small duffel bag, should be used in place of a purse. A purse can become contaminated when carried from house to house. The home care bag should not be placed on the floor or on the client's bed or table. It should be placed on clean pieces of paper which the family can provide. It should be put in an area close to where the client's care will be given. This area can be designated the *home care corner*. This is an excellent spot to keep any other supplies caregivers might need as they care for the client. These include gloves, care plans, education materials, and dressings and tape.

Spread of Infection

Medical asepsis refers to measures used to reduce and prevent the spread of pathogens. **Pathogens** are **microorganisms** that are capable of causing infection and disease. Medical asepsis is used in all healthcare settings. Preventing the spread of infection is important. To understand how to prevent disease, it is helpful to first know how it is spread. The chain of infection is a way of describing how disease is transmitted from one being to another. The six links in the chain of infection are as follows:

Link 1: The **causative agent** is a pathogenic microorganism that causes disease. Causative agents include bacteria, viruses, fungi, and parasites.

Link 2: A **reservoir** is where the pathogen lives and grows. Examples of reservoirs include the lungs, blood, and the large intestine.

Link 3: The **portal of exit** is any body opening on an infected person that allows pathogens to leave. These include the nose, mouth, eyes, or a cut in the skin.

Link 4: The **mode of transmission** describes how the pathogen travels. Transmission can occur through the air or through **direct contact** or **indirect contact**. The primary route of disease transmission within the healthcare setting is on the hands of healthcare workers.

Link 5: The **portal of entry** is any body opening on an uninfected person that allows pathogens to enter. These include the nose, mouth, eyes, and other mucous membranes, cuts in the skin, and cracked skin.

Link 6: A **susceptible host** is an uninfected person who could get sick. Examples include all healthcare workers and anyone in their care who is not already infected with that particular disease.

If one of the links in the chain of infection is broken, then the spread of infection is stopped.

Standard Precautions

The Centers for Disease Control and Prevention (CDC) (cdc.gov) is a government agency that issues information to protect the health of individuals and communities. In 1996, the CDC recommended a new infection prevention system to reduce the risk of contracting infectious diseases in healthcare settings. It has been updated since. There are two tiers of precautions within the infection prevention system: Standard Precautions and Transmission-Based Precautions.

Standard Precautions means treating all blood, body fluids, non-intact skin (like abrasions, pimples, or open sores), and **mucous membranes** (linings of mouth, nose, eyes, rectum, and genitals) as if they were infected. Body fluids include saliva, sputum (mucus coughed up), urine, feces, semen, vaginal secretions, pus or other wound drainage, and vomit. They do not include sweat.

Standard Precautions must be used with every client. This promotes safety. An HHA cannot tell by looking at clients if they have an **infectious** disease such as tuberculosis, hepatitis, or influenza.

Guidelines: Standard Precautions

G   **Wash your hands** before putting on gloves. Wash your hands immediately after removing gloves. Be careful not to touch clean objects with your used gloves.

G   **Wear gloves** if you may come into contact with blood; body fluids or secretions; broken skin, such as abrasions, acne, cuts, stitches or staples; or mucous membranes. Such contact occurs during mouth care; toilet assistance; perineal care; helping with a bedpan or urinal; ostomy care; cleaning up spills; cleaning basins, urinals, bedpans, and other containers that have held body fluids; and disposing of wastes.

G   **Remove gloves** immediately when finished with a procedure.

G   **Immediately wash all skin surfaces that have been contaminated** with blood and body fluids.

G   **Wear a disposable gown** that is resistant to body fluids if you may come into contact with blood or body fluids or when splashing or spraying blood or body fluids is likely.

G   **Wear a mask and protective goggles** if you may come into contact with blood or body fluids or when splashing or spraying blood or body fluids is likely.

G   **Wear gloves and use caution when handling razor blades, needles, and other sharps.** **Sharps** are needles or other sharp objects. Place sharps carefully in a biohazard container for sharps, which are hard, leakproof containers. They are clearly labeled and warn of the danger of the contents inside (Fig. 2-1).

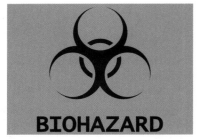

Fig. 2-1. This label indicates that the material is potentially infectious.

G   **Never attempt to recap needles or sharps after use.** You might stick yourself. Dispose of them in a biohazard container for sharps.

G   **Avoid nicks and cuts** when shaving clients.

G   **Carefully bag all contaminated supplies.** Dispose of them according to your agency's policy.

G   **Clearly label body fluids that are being saved for a specimen** with the client's name, date of birth, date, and a biohazard label. Keep them in a container with a lid.

G   **Dispose of contaminated wastes according to your agency's policy.**

HHAs use their hands constantly while they work. Microorganisms are on everything they touch. Handwashing is the single most important thing HHAs can do to prevent the spread of disease. The CDC has defined **hand hygiene** as washing hands with either plain or antiseptic soap and water or using alcohol-based hand rubs. Alcohol-based hand rubs (often called *hand sanitizers*) include gels, rinses, and foams that do not require the use of water.

Alcohol-based hand rubs have proven effective in reducing bacteria on the skin. However, they are not a substitute for proper handwashing. When hands are visibly soiled, they should be washed using **antimicrobial** soap and water. Once hands are clean, hand rubs can be used in addition to handwashing any time hands are not visibly soiled. When using a hand rub, the hands must be rubbed together until the product has completely dried. Hand lotion can help prevent dry, cracked skin.

HHAs should avoid wearing rings while working. Rings may increase the risk of contamination. Fingernails should be short, smooth, and clean. Artificial nails or extenders should not be worn because they harbor bacteria and increase the risk of contamination. HHAs should wash their hands at these times:

- When first arriving at a client's home
- Whenever hands are visibly soiled
- Before and after all contact with a client
- Before putting on gloves and after removing gloves
- After contact with any body fluids, mucous membranes, non-intact skin, or wound dressings
- After handling contaminated items
- Before and after making meals or working in the kitchen
- Before and after feeding a client
- Before getting clean linen
- Before reaching into the clean area of the supply bag
- After touching garbage or trash
- After picking up anything from the floor
- Before and after using the toilet
- After nose-blowing or coughing or sneezing into hands
- Before and after eating
- After smoking
- After touching areas on the body, such as the mouth, face, eyes, hair, ears, or nose

- After any contact with pets and after contact with pet care items
- Before leaving a client's home

Washing hands (hand hygiene)

Equipment: soap, paper towels

1. Turn on water at sink. Keep your clothes dry, because moisture breeds bacteria.

2. Wet hands and wrists thoroughly (Fig. 2-2).

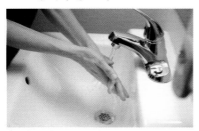

Fig. 2-2. Keeping arms angled downward, wet hands and wrists thoroughly.

3. Apply soap to your hands.

4. Keep your hands lower than your elbows and your fingertips down. Rub your hands together and fingers between each other to create a lather. Lather all surfaces of wrists, hands, and fingers, using friction for at least 20 seconds (Fig. 2-3).

5. Clean your nails by rubbing them in the palm of your hand.

6. Keep your hands lower than your elbows and your fingertips down. Being careful not to touch the sink, rinse thoroughly under running water. Rinse all surfaces of your wrists, hands, and fingers. Run water down from wrists to fingertips. Do not run water over unwashed arms down to clean hands.

7. Use a clean, dry paper towel to dry all surfaces of your hands, wrists, and fingers. Do not wipe towel on your unwashed forearms and then wipe clean hands. Dispose of towel into waste container without touching the container. If your hands touch the sink or wastebasket, start over.

8. Use a clean, dry paper towel to turn off the faucet (Fig. 2-4). Dispose of paper towel into waste container. Do not contaminate your hands by touching the surface of the sink or faucet.

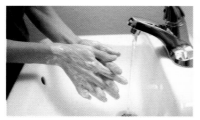

Fig. 2-3. Using friction for at least 20 seconds, lather all surfaces of fingers and hands.

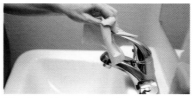

Fig. 2-4. Use a clean, dry paper towel to turn off faucet so that you do not contaminate your hands.

Personal Protective Equipment (PPE)

Personal protective equipment (PPE) is equipment that helps protect employees from serious injuries or illnesses resulting from contact with workplace hazards. Employers are responsible for giving HHAs the appropriate PPE to wear for client assignments.

Personal protective equipment includes gowns, masks, goggles, face shields, and gloves. Gowns protect the skin and/or clothing. Masks protect the mouth and nose. Goggles protect the eyes. Face shields protect the entire face—the eyes, mouth, and nose. Gloves protect the hands. Gloves are the PPE used most often by caregivers.

PPE must be worn if there is a chance the HHA could come into contact with body fluids, mucous membranes, or open wounds. HHAs must wear, or don, gowns, masks, goggles, and face shields when splashing or spraying of body fluids or blood could occur. When finished with a procedure, HHAs should remove, or doff, the gown as soon as possible and wash their hands.

Putting on (donning) gown and removing (doffing) gown

1. Wash your hands.

2. Open gown. Hold out in front of you and allow gown to open/unfold. Do not shake it (Fig. 2-5). Facing the back opening of the gown, place an arm through each sleeve.

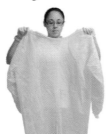

Fig. 2-5. Let the gown unfold without shaking it.

3. Fasten the neck opening.

4. Reach behind you. Pull the gown until it completely covers your clothing. Secure gown at waist (Fig. 2-6).

5. Use a gown only once and then remove and discard it. If gown becomes wet or soiled during care, remove it. Check clothing. Put on a new gown. The Occupational Safety and Health Administration (OSHA) requires non-permeable gowns—gowns that liquids cannot penetrate—when working in a bloody situation.

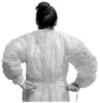

Fig. 2-6. Reaching behind you, secure the gown at the waist.

6. Put on your gloves after putting on gown. The cuffs of gloves should overlap the cuffs of the gown.

7. When removing a gown, remove and discard gloves properly (see procedure later in the chapter). Unfasten gown at neck and waist. Remove the gown without touching the outside of gown. Roll the dirty side in, while holding gown away from your body. Dispose of gown properly and wash your hands.

Masks should be worn when caring for clients with respiratory illnesses. They should also be worn when it is likely that contact with blood or body fluids will occur. HHAs must always change their masks between caring for different clients. The same mask should not be worn from one client to another. Goggles provide protection for the eyes. They are used when it is likely that blood or body fluids will be splashed or sprayed into the eye area or into the eyes.

Putting on (donning) mask and goggles

1. Wash your hands.

2. Pick up mask by top strings or elastic strap. Do not touch mask where it touches your face.

3. Pull elastic strap over your head, or if mask has strings, tie top strings first, then bottom strings. Do not wear a mask hanging from only the bottom tie or strap. Masks must always be dry or they must be replaced.

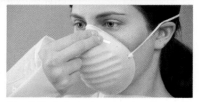

Fig. 2-7. Adjust the metal strip until the mask fits snugly around your nose.

4. Pinch the metal strip at the top of the mask (if part of mask) tightly around your nose so that it feels snug (Fig. 2-7).

5. Put on the goggles over your eyes or eyeglasses. Use the headband to secure them to your head. Make sure they are on snugly.

6. Put on gloves after putting on mask and goggles.

When additional skin protection is needed (if part of agency policy), a face shield can be used as a substitute for wearing a mask or goggles.

Agencies have specific policies regarding when to wear gloves. HHAs must learn and follow these rules. Gloves must always be worn for the following tasks:

*   Any time an HHA might come into contact with blood or any body fluid, open wounds, or mucous membranes

*   When performing or helping with mouth care or care of any mucous membrane

- When performing or helping with **perineal care** (care of the genitals and anal area)

- When performing personal care on non-intact skin—skin that is broken by abrasions, cuts, rashes, acne, pimples, lesions, surgical incisions, or boils

- When assisting with personal care when the HHA has open sores or cuts on her hands

- When shaving a client

- When disposing of soiled bed linens, gowns, dressings, and pads

- When touching surfaces or equipment that is either visibly contaminated or may be contaminated

Clean, non-sterile gloves are generally adequate. They may be latex, vinyl, or nitrile; however, some people are allergic to latex. An HHA should let the supervisor know if she is allergic to latex. Alternative gloves will be provided. An HHA should also tell the supervisor if she has dry, cracked, or broken skin. Non-intact areas should be covered with bandages or gauze before putting on gloves. Disposable gloves can only be worn once. They may not be washed or reused. Gloves should be changed immediately if they become soiled, torn, or damaged. Gloves should also be changed before contact with mucous membranes or broken skin. After removing gloves, the HHA should wash her hands before donning new gloves.

Putting on (donning) gloves

1. **Wash your hands.**

2. **If you are right-handed, slide one glove on your left hand (reverse if left-handed).**

3. **Using your gloved hand, slide the other hand into the second glove.**

4. **Interlace fingers to smooth out folds and create a comfortable fit.**

5. **Carefully look for tears, holes, or spots. Replace the glove if necessary.**

6. **If wearing a gown, pull the cuff of the gloves over the sleeves of the gown (Fig. 2-8).**

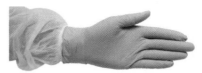

Fig. 2-8. Adjust gloves until they are pulled up over the sleeves of the gown.

Gloves should be removed promptly after use, and the HHA should wash her hands. Gloves are worn to protect the skin from becoming contaminated. After giving care, gloves are contaminated. If the HHA opens a door with a gloved hand, the doorknob becomes contaminated. Later, anyone who opens the door with an ungloved hand will be touching a contaminated surface. Before touching surfaces, the HHA must remove gloves and wash her hands. Afterward, new gloves can be donned if needed.

Removing (doffing) gloves

1. Touch only the outside of one glove. With one gloved hand, grasp the other glove at the palm and pull the glove off (Fig. 2-9).

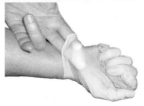

Fig. 2-10. Reach inside glove at wrist, without touching any part of the outside of glove.

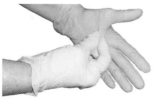

Fig. 2-9. Grasp the glove at the palm and pull it off.

2. With the fingertips of your gloved hand, hold the glove you just removed. With your ungloved hand, slip two fingers underneath cuff of the remaining glove at wrist. Do not touch any part of the outside of glove (Fig. 2-10).

3. Pull down, turning this glove inside out and over the first glove as you remove it.

4. You should now be holding one glove from its clean inner side. The other glove should be inside it.

5. Drop both gloves into the proper container without contaminating yourself.

6. Wash your hands.

Special Precautions

Spills, especially those involving blood, body fluids, or glass, can pose a serious risk of infection or injury. Hospitals and long-term care settings have special types of floors and specific solutions they use for spills. In the home, such products may not be available. HHAs should read the labels of cleaning products carefully. Certain precautions may need to be taken with their use. For example, they may contain bleach that could take the color out of a carpet as well as removing the stain or spill.

Guidelines: Cleaning Spills Involving Blood, Body Fluids, or Glass

G When blood or body fluids are spilled, put on gloves before starting to clean up the spill. Industrial-strength gloves are best.

G If blood or body fluids are spilled on a hard surface such as a linoleum floor or countertop, clean immediately using a solution of one part household bleach to nine parts water. You can mix the solution in a bucket and with gloves on, wipe up the spill with rags or paper towels dipped in the solution. Be careful not to spill bleach or bleach solution on clothes, carpets, or bedding. It can discolor and damage fabrics. Your employer may provide you with special products for cleaning spills.

G   If blood or body fluids are spilled on fabrics such as carpets, bedding, or clothes, do not use bleach to clean the spill. Commercial disinfectants that do not contain bleach are available. If you have no disinfectant, wear gloves and wipe spills. Then use soap and water to clean the area. Clean carpet with regular carpet cleaner. Use gloves to load soiled bedding or clothes into the washing machine and add color-safe bleach to the washer with the laundry detergent.

G   Do not pick up any pieces of broken glass, no matter how large, with your hands. Use a dustpan and broom or other tools.

G   Waste containing broken glass, blood, or body fluids should be properly bagged. Waste containing blood or body fluids may need to be placed in a special biohazard waste bag and disposed of separately from household trash. Follow your agency's policy.

Transmission-Based Precautions

Transmission-Based Precautions are used when caring for persons who are infected or suspected of being infected with a disease. When ordered, these precautions are used **in addition** to Standard Precautions. These precautions will always be listed in the care plan and on the assignment sheet. Following these precautions promotes the HHA's safety, as well as the safety of others.

There are three categories of Transmission-Based Precautions: Airborne Precautions, Droplet Precautions, and Contact Precautions. The category used depends on the disease and how it spreads to other people. They may also be used in combination for diseases that have multiple routes of transmission.

Airborne Precautions

Airborne Precautions are used for diseases that are transmitted, or spread, through the air after being expelled. The pathogens are so small that they can attach to moisture in the air. They remain floating for some time. For certain care, HHAs may be required to wear special masks, such as N95 or high efficiency particulate air (HEPA) masks, to avoid being infected. Airborne diseases include tuberculosis, measles, and chickenpox.

Droplet Precautions

Droplet Precautions are used for diseases that are spread by droplets in the air. Droplets normally do not travel more than six feet. Coughing, sneezing, talking, laughing, or suctioning can spread droplets. Droplet Precautions include wearing a face mask during care and restricting visits from uninfected people. HHAs should cover their noses and mouths with a tissue when they sneeze or cough. They should ask others to do the same. Used tissues should be disposed of in the nearest waste container; they should not be placed in a pocket for later use. If a tissue is not available, HHAs should cough or sneeze into their upper sleeve or elbow, not their hands. They should wash their hands immediately afterward. An example of a droplet disease is mumps.

Contact Precautions

Contact Precautions are used when there is a risk of spreading or contracting a microorganism from touching an infected object or person. Conjunctivitis (pink eye) and *Clostridium difficile* (*C. diff*) are examples of situations that require Contact Precautions. Transmission can occur with skin-to-skin contact during transfers or bathing. Contact Precautions include wearing PPE and client isolation. They require washing hands with antimicrobial soap. They also require not touching infected surfaces with ungloved hands or uninfected surfaces with contaminated gloves.

Guidelines: Isolation Procedures

G When they are indicated, Transmission-Based Precautions are always used **in addition** to Standard Precautions.

G Wash plates and utensils thoroughly in very hot water with antibacterial soap. Bleach may need to be added to the water. Follow agency policy. Family members should use separate dishes and utensils.

G Wear disposable gloves when handling soiled laundry. Bag laundry in the client's room and carry it to the laundry area in the bag. Wash the client's laundry separately. Use hot water and detergent.

G The amount of non-disposable equipment brought into the home should be limited. If some care equipment cannot remain in the home (for example, your stethoscope), clean and disinfect items before taking them from the home.

G Use a bleach solution (one part bleach to nine parts water) to clean up spills of blood or body fluids and to disinfect surfaces.

G Clean and disinfect frequently-touched surfaces and equipment, such as tables, bedside commodes, television remotes, canes, wheelchairs, and doorknobs at least daily.

G   Clients need to feel that caregivers understand what they are going through. Listen to what clients are saying. Reassure them and explain why these steps are being taken.

MRSA

MRSA stands for methicillin-resistant *Staphylococcus aureus*. *Staphylococcus aureus* is an antibiotic-resistant infection often acquired in healthcare facilities. This type of MRSA is also known as *HA-MRSA*, which stands for hospital-associated MRSA. Community-associated methicillin-resistant *Staphylococcus aureus* (CA-MRSA) is a type of MRSA infection that occurs in people who have not recently been admitted to healthcare facilities and who have no past diagnosis of MRSA. Often CA-MRSA manifests as skin infections, such as pimples or boils.

MRSA is almost always spread by direct physical contact with infected people or objects. This means if a person has MRSA on his skin, especially on the hands, and touches another person, he may spread MRSA. Spread also occurs through indirect contact by touching objects, such as sheets or wound dressings, contaminated by a person who has MRSA.

HHAs can help prevent MRSA by practicing proper hygiene. Handwashing, using soap and warm water, is the single most important measure to control the spread of MRSA. Cuts and abrasions should be kept clean and covered with a proper dressing (e.g., bandage) until healed. Contact with other people's wounds or material that is contaminated from wounds should be avoided.

Several state and federal government agencies have guidelines and laws concerning infection prevention. **The Occupational Safety and Health Administration** (**OSHA**) (osha.gov) requires employers to provide for the safety of their employees through rules and suggested guidelines. The Centers for Disease Control issues guidelines for healthcare workers to follow on the job. Some of the infection prevention requirements for employers and employees are listed below.

Employers' responsibilities for infection prevention include the following:

- Establish infection prevention procedures and an **exposure control plan** to protect workers

- Provide continuing in-service education on infection prevention, including airborne and **bloodborne pathogens** and updates on any new safety standards

- Have written procedures to follow should an exposure occur, including medical treatment and plans to prevent similar exposures
- Provide PPE for employees to use and train them on when and how to properly use it
- Provide free hepatitis B vaccinations for all employees

Employees' responsibilities for infection prevention include the following:

- Follow Standard Precautions
- Follow all agency policies and procedures
- Follow client care plans and assignments
- Use provided PPE as indicated or as appropriate
- Take advantage of the free hepatitis B vaccination
- Immediately report any exposure to infection
- Participate in annual education programs covering infection prevention

Safety and Body Mechanics

Principles of Body Mechanics

Back strain or injury is a serious problem for home health aides. Using proper body mechanics is an important step in preventing back strain and injury. **Body mechanics** is the way the parts of the body work together when a person moves. Understanding some basic principles of body mechanics helps promote safety.

Alignment. When standing, sitting, or lying down, the body should be in alignment. This means that the two sides of the body are mirror images of each other, with body parts lined up naturally. A person can maintain correct body alignment when lifting or carrying an object by keeping it close to his body. His feet and body should be pointed in the direction he is moving. He should avoid twisting at the waist.

Base of support. The base of support is the foundation that supports an object. The feet are the body's base of support. The wider the support, the more stable a person will be. Standing with legs apart allows for a greater base of support. This is more stable than standing with feet together.

Center of gravity. The center of gravity in the body is the point where the most weight is concentrated. This point will depend on the position of the body. When a person stands, weight is centered in the pelvis. A low center of gravity gives a more stable base of support. Bending the knees when lifting an object lowers the pelvis and, therefore, lowers a person's center of gravity. This gives more stability and makes the person less likely to fall or strain the working muscles.

Guidelines: Using Proper Body Mechanics

G   Assess the situation first. Clear the path. Remove any obstacles.

G   Use both arms and hands to lift, push, or carry objects.

G   When lifting a heavy object from the floor, spread your feet shoulder-width apart and bend your knees. Use the strong, large muscles in your thighs, upper arms, and shoulders to lift the object. Raise your body and the object together.

G   Hold objects close to you when lifting or carrying them. This keeps the object closer to your center of gravity and base of support.

G   Push or slide objects rather than lifting them.

G   Avoid bending and reaching as much as possible. Move or position furniture so that you do not have to bend or reach.

G   If you are making an adjustable bed, adjust the height to a safe working level, usually waist high. Avoid bending at the waist.

G   When a task requires bending, use a good stance. Bend your knees to lower yourself, rather than bending from the waist. This uses the big muscles in your legs and thighs rather than the smaller muscles in your back.

G   Do not twist when you are lifting or moving an object. Instead, turn your whole body. Pivot your feet instead of twisting at the waist. Your feet should point toward what you are lifting or moving.

G   Talk to the client before moving him. Let him know what you will do so he can help if possible. Agree on a signal, such as counting to three. Lift or move on three so that everyone moves together.

G   To help a client sit up, stand up, or walk, place your feet shoulder-width apart. Put one foot in front of the other, and bend your knees. Your upper body should stay upright and in alignment. Do this whenever you have to support a client's weight.

G   Never try to catch a falling client. If a client falls, assist him to the floor. If you try to reverse a fall in progress, you could injure yourself and/or the client.

G   Report any task you feel you cannot safely perform to your supervisor. Never try to lift an object or a client that you feel you cannot handle.

Here are several strategies that can help you apply good body mechanics in the home:

G **Have the right tools for the job**. For example, if you cannot reach an object on a high shelf, use a step stool rather than climbing on a counter or straining to reach.

G **Have footrests and pillows available**. Tasks that require standing for long periods can be more comfortable if you rest one foot on a footrest. This position flexes the muscles in the lower back and keeps the spine in alignment. When sitting, using a footrest allows for a more comfortable leg position. Crossing the legs disrupts alignment and should be avoided. Using pillows can make any chair more comfortable. Use pillows behind the back to keep the back straight.

G **Keep tools, supplies, and clutter off the floor**. Keep frequently-used items on shelves or counters where they can be easily reached without lifting. Keeping things organized will also help you find what you need without straining.

G **Whenever you can sit to do a job, do so**. Chopping vegetables, folding clothes, and other tasks can be done easily while sitting. For jobs like scouring the bathtub, kneel or use a low stool. Avoid bending at the waist.

G **Use gait or transfer belts when assisting clients with ambulation or transfers**. Section IV contains the correct procedures for safely assisting clients with ambulation and transfers.

Accident Prevention

Falls: Falls are among the most common home accidents. They can be caused by an unsafe environment, loss of abilities, diseases, advanced age, and medications. Falls are particularly common among the elderly. Older people are often more seriously injured by falls because their bones are more fragile. HHAs must be especially alert to the risk of falls with elderly clients. All falls must be reported to the supervisor, even if the client says he is fine.

These factors increase the risk of falls:

- Clutter
- Throw rugs
- Exposed electrical cords
- Slippery or wet floors
- Uneven floors or stairs
- Poor lighting

Personal conditions that raise the risk of falls include medications, loss of vision, gait or balance problems, weakness, paralysis, and disorientation. **Disorientation** means confusion about person, place, or time.

Guidelines: Preventing Falls

G   Clear all walkways of clutter, trash, throw rugs, and cords.

G   Avoid waxing floors, and use non-skid mats where appropriate.

G   Have clients wear non-skid shoes. Make sure shoelaces are tied.

G   Clients should wear clothing that is not too long.

G   Keep personal items that are used often close to the client.

G   Immediately clean up spills on the floor.

G   Mark uneven flooring or stairs with tape of a contrasting color to indicate a hazard.

G   Improve lighting where needed.

G   Lock wheels and move footrests out of the way before helping clients into or out of wheelchairs.

G   Return adjustable beds to their lowest position when you have finished with care.

G   Offer trips to the bathroom often. Respond to clients' requests for bathroom assistance promptly.

Burns/Scalds: Burns can be caused by dry heat (e.g., a hot iron, stove, other electrical appliances), wet heat (e.g., hot water or other liquids, steam), or chemicals (e.g., lye, acids). Small children, older adults, or people with loss of sensation (such as from paralysis or diabetes) are at greatest risk of burns. Scalds are burns caused by hot liquids. It takes five seconds or less for a serious burn to occur when the temperature of a liquid is 140°F. Coffee, tea, and other hot drinks are usually served at 160°F to 180°F. Preventing burns is very important.

Guidelines: Preventing Burns and Scalds

G   Roll up sleeves and avoid loose clothing when working at the stove.

G   Check that the stove and appliances are off when you leave.

G   Suggest that the hot water heater be set lower than normal. It should be set at 120°F to 130°F to avoid burns from scalding tap water.

G   Always check water temperature with a bath thermometer or on your wrist before using.

G   Check temperatures of liquids on your wrist before serving.

G   Keep space heaters away from clients' beds, chairs, and draperies. Never allow space heaters to be used in the bathroom.

G   Report frayed electrical cords or appliances that look unsafe immediately. Do not use these appliances.

G   Let clients know you are about to pour or set down a hot liquid.

G   Pour hot drinks away from clients. Keep hot drinks and liquids away from edges of tables. Put lids on them.

G   Make sure clients are sitting down before serving hot drinks.

Poisoning: Homes contain many harmful substances that should not be swallowed. These include cleaning products, paints, medicines, toiletries, and glues. These products should be locked away from confused clients, clients with limited vision, and children. Clients who have a diminished sense of taste or smell due to stroke or head injury might eat spoiled food. Clients with dementia may hide food and let it spoil in closets, drawers, or other places. HHAs should check the refrigerator and cabinets frequently for foods that are moldy, sour, or spoiled. They should investigate any odors they notice. The number for the Poison Control Center should be posted by the telephone.

Cuts: Cuts typically occur in the kitchen or bathroom. Sharp objects, including knives, peelers, graters, food processor blades, scissors, nail clippers, and razors must be kept out of the reach of children. Sharp objects should also be locked away if there is a confused client in the home. When preparing food, an HHA should cut away from herself, use a cutting board, and keep her fingers out of the way. She must also know proper first aid for cuts.

Choking: Choking can occur when eating, drinking, or taking medication. Babies and young children who put objects in their mouths are at great risk of choking. People who are weak, ill, or unconscious may choke on their own saliva. A person's tongue can also become swollen and obstruct his airway. Babies and small children should never have access to small objects. Clients who have trouble with utensils and children who are too young to manage utensils need their food cut into bite-sized pieces. Pillows, small toys, and other objects should never be placed in a crib with an infant. To prevent sudden infant death syndrome (SIDS), infants should be always be placed on their backs for sleeping. Clients should eat in as upright a position as possible to avoid choking. Clients with swallowing problems may have a special diet with liquids thickened to the consistency of honey or syrup. Thickened liquids are easier to swallow. Section VI has more information on thickened liquids.

Fire: To guard against fire, HHAs should follow these guidelines:

Guidelines: Reducing Fire Hazards and Responding to Fires

G   Roll up clients' sleeves and avoid loose clothing when clients may be cooking or around the stove.

G   Store potholders, dish towels, and other flammable kitchen items away from the stove.

G   Never store cookies, candy, or other items that may attract children above or near the stove.

G   Discourage careless smoking and smoking in bed. If clients must smoke, check to be sure that cigarettes are extinguished when they are finished. Empty ashtrays frequently. Before emptying ashtrays, make sure there are no hot ashes or hot matches in them.

G   Stay in or near the kitchen when anything is cooking or baking.

G   Do not leave the dryer on when you leave the house. Lint can catch fire. Empty lint traps each time you use the dryer.

G   Turn off space heaters when no one is home or everyone is asleep.

G   Check monthly to see that smoke alarms are working. Replace batteries when needed.

G   Have fire extinguishers on hand. Every home should have a fire extinguisher in the kitchen. Check that the homes you work in have fire extinguishers that have not expired. Know where the fire extinguisher is stored and how to operate it. The PASS acronym will help you understand how to use it:

Pull the pin.

Aim at the base of the fire when spraying.

Squeeze the handle.

Sweep back and forth at the base of the fire.

G   In case of fire, the RACE acronym is a good rule to follow:

Remove clients from danger.

Activate 911.

Contain fire if possible.

Extinguish, or call fire department to extinguish.

In addition, follow these guidelines for helping clients and family members exit the home safely:

G   Remain calm.

G   Be sure all family members know how to exit in case of fire, and have a designated meeting place outside the home.

G   Do not try to put out a large fire. All household members should leave the house and call the fire department immediately.

G   If windows or doors have locking bars, keep keys in the lock or nearby. Mark windows of children's rooms with stickers that indicate a child sleeps in the room.

G   Remove anything blocking a window or door that could be used as a fire exit.

G   Stay low in a room to escape a fire.

G   Do not use elevators.

G   If door is closed, check for heat coming from it before opening it. If the door or doorknob feels hot to the touch, it is best to stay in the room if there is no safe exit. Plug the doorway (use wet towels or clothing) to prevent smoke from entering. Stay in the room until help arrives.

G   Use the "stop, drop, and roll" fire safety technique to extinguish a fire on clothing or hair. Stop running or stay still. Drop to the ground, lying down if possible. Roll on the ground to try to extinguish the flames.

G   Use a damp covering over the face to reduce smoke inhalation.

G   After leaving the home, move away from it, to the designated meeting place.

Travel Safety

Because HHAs may be driving to and from clients' homes, they must be careful to protect themselves from possible dangers:

Guidelines: Traveling Safely

G   Plan your route. Driving while trying to look at a map can be very dangerous. Study the directions before beginning. If you are using a phone or other GPS device for navigation, activate the voice instructions so you do not have to look at the device while you drive.

G   Minimize distractions. Paying attention to the road can help avoid accidents. Keep your eyes on the road and your hands on the steering wheel. If music is distracting, do not listen to it in the car. Do not talk on your cell phone. Do not send or read text messages or emails while driving.

G   Use turn signals. Using turn signals lets other drivers know what you are planning to do. Always use turn signals when preparing to turn or change lanes.

G   Use caution when backing up. Many accidents occur when drivers back up. When you back up, look around carefully. Turn your head to both sides and look behind your car.

G   Drive at a safe speed. Follow speed limits to be sure you are not driving too fast. Road conditions such as ice or heavy rain may make it necessary to drive at a slower speed.

G   Always wear your seat belt. Although it may not help you avoid an accident, it will certainly help protect you if an accident occurs.

G   Keep your driver's license, valid car insurance, and proof of registration with you in case you are in an accident or stopped by police.

If an HHA's assignment takes her to an area where crime is a problem, she should use caution. If she is using public transportation, she should be alert at all times.

Guidelines: Staying Safe in High-Crime Areas

G   Park in well-lit areas as close as possible to the home you are visiting.

G   Try to leave valuables at home when you must work in a dangerous area.

G   Hold your home care bag tightly, close to your body.

G   Lock your car and do not leave any valuables in it.

G   Walk confidently. Look as though you know where you are going (Fig. 2-11).

G   Carry a whistle so you can make a loud noise to startle an attacker and get help.

G   Carry your keys in your hand to unlock your car as soon as you arrive. If necessary, you can also use them as a weapon.

G   Do not sit in your car, even with the doors locked. Drive away as soon as you reach your car.

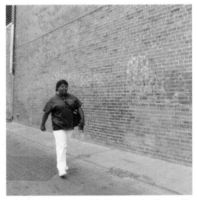

Fig. 2-11. *Be cautious but look confident if you enter a high-crime area.*

G   Try to avoid unsafe areas after dark.

G   If you are concerned about your safety in a particular area, leave the area immediately. Contact your supervisor.

G   Do not approach a home where strangers are hanging around. Go to your car and drive to a safe area. Use your cell phone or the nearest phone in a safe area, and call your supervisor.

G   Call your client before you visit so he or she knows approximately when to expect you.

G   Never enter a vacant home.

G   If necessary, ask your supervisor to arrange for an escort or another care provider to go with you.

G   Be sure someone knows your schedule. Call the office at the end of your work day.

Emergencies

Medical Emergencies

Medical emergencies may be the result of accidents or sudden illnesses. This section discusses what to do in a medical emergency. Heart attacks, stroke, diabetic emergencies, choking, automobile accidents, and gunshot wounds are all medical emergencies. Falls, burns, and cuts can also be emergencies. In an emergency, responders should remain calm, act quickly, and communicate clearly. These steps will help:

Assess the situation. The responder should try to find out what has happened. She must make sure she is not in danger. She should notice the time.

Assess the victim. The responder should ask the injured or ill person what has happened. If the person is unable to respond, he may be unconscious. Tapping the person and asking if he is all right helps to determine if a person is conscious. The responder should speak loudly and use the person's name if she knows it. If there is no response, she should assume the person is unconscious. This is an emergency situation. She should call for help right away or send someone else to call.

If a person is conscious and able to speak, then he is breathing and has a pulse. The responder should talk with him about what happened. She should get the person's permission to touch him. The person should be checked for the following: severe bleeding, changes in consciousness, irregular breathing, unusual color or feel to the skin, swollen places on the body, medical alert tags, and anything the person says is painful. If any of these exist, professional medical help may be needed. The HHA should always get help before doing anything else.

If the injured or ill person is conscious, he may be frightened. The responder should listen to the person and tell him what is being done to help him. A calm and confident response will help reassure him.

When an HHA is in doubt about calling for help, she should call. If she is alone, she should make the call herself by dialing 911. If she is not alone, she should shout for help and have someone make the call for her and then return to assist her. After calling 911, the HHA should notify her supervisor. When calling emergency services, a responder should be prepared to give the following information:

- The phone number and address of the emergency, including exact directions or landmarks if necessary
- The person's condition, including any known medical background
- The responder's name and position
- Details of any first aid being given

The dispatcher may need other information or may want to give other instructions. The HHA should not hang up the phone until the dispatcher hangs up or tells her to hang up. If the HHA is in a home, she should unlock the front door so emergency personnel can get in when they arrive.

If the person is breathing, has a normal pulse, is responsive, and is not bleeding severely, calling emergency services may not be necessary. If a client has fallen, been burned, or cut himself but the damage seems to be minor, the HHA should call her supervisor. She should let the person answering the phone know that she is with a client and that an accident has occurred. If her supervisor is not available, another member of the care team may be able to help.

Once the emergency is over, the HHA will need to document it in her notes and complete an incident report. It is important for her to include as many details as possible and report only facts. Knowing what information must be documented will help the HHA remember the important facts. Documenting emergencies accurately is very important.

First aid is emergency care given immediately to an injured person. **Cardiopulmonary resuscitation** (**CPR**) refers to the medical procedures used when a person's heart or lungs have stopped working. CPR is used until medical help arrives. Quick action is necessary. CPR must be started immediately. Only properly trained people should perform CPR. Employers often arrange for HHAs to be trained in CPR. If not, the HHA can contact the American Heart Association (heart.org) or Red Cross (redcross.org) for more information. CPR is an important skill to learn.

If a person is not trained, he or she should not attempt to perform CPR. Performing CPR incorrectly can further injure a person.

Choking

When something is blocking the tube through which air enters the lungs, the person has an obstructed airway. When people are choking, they usually put their hands to their throats (Fig 2-12). As long as a person can speak, breathe, or cough, the HHA should only encourage her to cough as forcefully as possible to get the object out. The HHA should stay with the person until she stops choking or can no longer speak, breathe, or cough. If a person can no longer speak, breathe, or cough, the HHA should call 911 and return to the person. Time is of extreme importance.

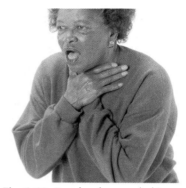

Fig. 2-12. *People who are choking usually put their hands to their throats.*

Abdominal thrusts are a method of attempting to remove an object from the airway of someone who is choking. These thrusts work to remove the blockage upward, out of the throat. The HHA should make sure the person needs help before starting to give abdominal thrusts. She must show signs of a severely obstructed airway. These signs include poor air exchange, an increase in trouble breathing, silent coughing, blue-tinged (cyanotic) skin, or inability to speak, breathe, or cough. The HHA should ask, "Are you choking? I know what to do. Can I help you?" If the client nods her head, "Yes," she has a severe airway obstruction and needs immediate help. The HHA should begin giving abdominal thrusts. This procedure should never be performed on a person who is not choking.

Performing abdominal thrusts for the conscious person

1. **Stand behind the person. Bring your arms under her arms. Wrap your arms around the person's waist.**

2. **Make a fist with one hand. Place the flat, thumb side of the fist against the person's abdomen, above the navel but below the breastbone.**

3. **Grasp the fist with your other hand. Pull both hands toward you and up, quickly and forcefully.**

4. **Repeat until the object is pushed out or the person loses consciousness.**

5. **Report and document the incident properly.**

Insulin Reaction and Diabetic Ketoacidosis

Insulin reaction, or hypoglycemia, can result from either too much insulin or too little food. It occurs when insulin is given, and the person skips a meal or does not eat all the food required. Even when a regular amount of food is eaten, physical activity may rapidly absorb the food. This causes too much insulin to be in the body. Vomiting and diarrhea may also lead to insulin reaction in people with diabetes.

The first signs of insulin reaction include feeling weak or different, nervousness, dizziness, and perspiration (see list below for further signs). These signal that the client needs food in a form that can be rapidly absorbed. A lump of sugar, a hard candy, or a small glass of juice should be consumed right away. A diabetic should always have a quick source of sugar handy. The supervisor should be notified if the client has shown signs of insulin reaction. Other signs and symptoms include the following:

- Hunger
- Weakness
- Rapid pulse
- Headache
- Low blood pressure
- Cold, clammy skin
- Confusion
- Trembling
- Nervousness
- Blurred vision
- Numbness of the lips and tongue
- Unconsciousness

Diabetic ketoacidosis (DKA), or hyperglycemia, is caused by having too little insulin. It can result from undiagnosed diabetes, going without insulin or not taking enough, eating too much, not getting enough exercise, infection, or physical or emotional stress. The signs of the onset of diabetic ketoacidosis include increased thirst or urination, abdominal pain, deep or labored breathing, and breath that smells sweet or fruity (see list below for further signs). The supervisor should be notified immediately if the client has shown signs of diabetic ketoacidosis. Other signs and symptoms include the following:

- Hunger
- Headache
- Weakness

- Rapid, weak pulse
- Low blood pressure
- Dry skin
- Flushed cheeks
- Drowsiness
- Nausea and vomiting
- Air hunger, or client gasping for air and being unable to catch his breath
- Unconsciousness

Section V contains more information about diabetes.

CVA or Stroke

Cerebrovascular accident (CVA), or stroke, occurs when blood supply to a part of the brain is blocked or a blood vessel leaks or ruptures within the brain. A quick response to a suspected stroke is critical. Tests and treatment need to be given within a short time of the stroke's onset. Early treatment may be able to reduce the severity of the stroke.

A transient ischemic attack (TIA) is a warning sign of a CVA. It is the result of a temporary lack of oxygen in the brain. Symptoms may last up to 24 hours. They include difficulty speaking, weakness on one side of the body, temporary loss of vision, and numbness or tingling. These symptoms should not be ignored. They should be reported to the supervisor immediately. These are also signs that a CVA is occurring:

- Facial numbness, weakness, or drooping, especially on one side
- Arm or leg numbness or weakness, especially on one side
- Slurred speech or inability to speak
- Use of inappropriate words
- Inability to understand spoken or written words
- Redness in the face
- Noisy breathing
- Dizziness
- Blurred vision
- Trouble walking, loss of balance
- Ringing in the ears
- Severe headache
- Nausea or vomiting
- Seizures

- Loss of bowel and bladder control
- Paralysis on one side of the body
- Elevated blood pressure
- Slow pulse rate
- Loss of consciousness

In addition to the symptoms listed above, women may have these symptoms:

- Pain in the face, arms, and legs
- Hiccups
- Weakness
- Chest pain
- Shortness of breath
- Palpitations

F.A.S.T.

The acronym **F.A.S.T.** can be used as a way to remember the sudden signs that a stroke is occurring. **(F)ace**: Is one side of the face drooping? Is it numb? Ask the person to smile. Is the smile uneven? **(A)rms**: Is one arm numb or weak? Ask the person to raise both arms. Check to see if one arm drifts downward. **(S)peech**: Is the person's speech slurred? Is the person unable to speak? Can the person be understood? Ask the person to repeat a simple sentence and see if the sentence is repeated correctly. **(T)ime**: Time is of the utmost importance when responding to a stroke. If the person shows any of the symptoms listed above, call 911 immediately. Websites for the American Stroke Association (strokeassociation.org) and The National Stroke Association (stroke.org) have more information. *Special Conditions* in Section V of this textbook contains more information on strokes.

Myocardial Infarction or Heart Attack

Myocardial infarction (**MI**), or heart attack, occurs when the heart muscle itself does not receive enough oxygen because blood vessels are blocked. A myocardial infarction is an emergency that can result in serious heart damage or death. The following are signs and symptoms of MI:

- Sudden, severe pain in the chest, usually on the left side or in the center, behind the breastbone
- Pain or discomfort in other areas of the body, such as one or both arms, the back, neck, jaw, or stomach

- Indigestion or heartburn
- Nausea and vomiting
- **Dyspnea**, or difficulty breathing
- Dizziness
- Bluish or gray (**cyanotic**) skin, indicating lack of oxygen
- Perspiration
- Cold and clammy skin
- Weak and irregular pulse rate
- Low blood pressure
- Anxiety and a sense of doom
- Denial of a heart problem

The pain of a heart attack is commonly described as a crushing, pressing, squeezing, stabbing, piercing pain, or, "like someone is sitting on my chest." The pain may go down the inside of the left arm. A person may also feel it in the neck and/or in the jaw. The pain usually does not go away.

As with men, women's most common symptom is chest pain or pressure. Women, though, can have heart attacks without chest pressure. Women are more likely to have shortness of breath, pressure or pain in the lower chest or upper abdomen, dizziness, lightheadedness, fainting, pressure in the upper back, or extreme fatigue. Some women's symptoms seem more flu-like, and women are more likely to deny that they are having a heart attack. HHAs must take immediate action if a client has any of these symptoms.

Responding to a heart attack

1. **Call or have someone call emergency services. Call your supervisor.**

2. **Place the person in a comfortable position. Encourage him to rest, and reassure him that you will not leave him alone.**

3. **Loosen clothing around the person's neck (Fig. 2-13).**

4. **Do not give the person liquids or food.**

5. **Monitor the person's breathing and pulse. If the person stops breathing or has no pulse,** **perform CPR if you are trained to do so.**

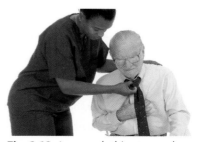

Fig. 2-13. Loosen clothing around the person's neck if you suspect he is having a heart attack.

6. **Stay with the person until help arrives.**

7. **Report and document the incident properly.**

Section V contains more information about heart attacks.

Disaster Guidelines

Disasters can include fire, flood, earthquake, hurricane, tornado, or severe weather. Manmade dangers, such as acts of terrorism or bomb threats, are also considered disasters. Home health aides need to be skilled and professional when a disaster occurs. Each agency has a local and area-specific disaster plan, and HHAs will be trained on these plans. They should pay close attention to instructions.

During disasters, agencies may rely on local or state management groups and the American Red Cross to assume responsibility for the ill and disabled.

Guidelines: Disasters

The following guidelines apply in any disaster situation:

G   Remain calm.

G   Use the internet to stay informed, or keep the television or radio tuned to a local station to get the latest information.

G   If a disaster is forecast (for example, a tornado or hurricane), be ready. Wear appropriate clothing and shoes. Have family members dressed and ready in case evacuation is necessary.

G   Stay in contact with your supervisor or others if possible. Let someone know where you are, what conditions exist, and where you will go if you must evacuate.

G   Locate disaster supplies. Ideally, a disaster supply kit should meet your needs for at least three days. It should be assembled before disaster strikes and should include the following:

- A three-day supply of water (one gallon per person per day) and food that will not spoil

- One change of clothing and footwear per person and one blanket or sleeping bag per person

- A first aid kit that includes your family's prescription medications

- Emergency tools, including a battery-powered radio, flashlight, and plenty of extra batteries

- An extra set of car keys and a credit card, cash, or debit card

- Sanitation supplies
- Special items for infant, elderly, or disabled family members
- An extra pair of eyeglasses
- Important family documents in a waterproof container

In addition, you will be required to apply specific guidelines for the area in which you work. For example, an HHA working where hurricanes are prevalent, such as Florida, needs to know the guidelines for hurricane preparedness, as well as for storms and fires. The following general guidelines are organized by the type of disaster.

Tornadoes

G Seek shelter inside, ideally in a steel-framed or concrete building.

G Stay away from windows.

G Stand in the hallway or in a basement, or take cover under heavy furniture.

G Do not stay in a mobile home or trailer.

G Lie as flat as possible.

Lightning

If outdoors, follow these guidelines:

G Avoid the largest objects, such as trees, and avoid open spaces.

G Stay out of the water.

G Seek shelter in buildings.

G Stay away from metal fences, doors, or other objects.

G Avoid holding metal objects, such as golf clubs, in your hands.

G Stay in automobiles.

G It is safe to perform CPR on lightning victims if you are trained to do so; they carry no electricity.

If indoors, follow these guidelines:

G Stay inside and away from open doors and windows.

G Avoid the use of electrical equipment, such as hair dryers and televisions.

Floods

G Fill the bathtub with fresh water.

G Board up windows.

G Evacuate if advised to do so.

G Check the fuel level in automobiles. Make sure there is enough fuel to last through an evacuation if one becomes necessary.

G Have a portable battery-operated radio, flashlight, and cooking equipment available.

G Do not drink water or eat food that has been contaminated with flood water.

G Do not handle electrical equipment.

G Do not turn off gas yourself. Ask the gas company to turn off the gas.

Blackouts

G Ask your client where the emergency supplies are kept. Take prompt action to keep calm and provide light.

G Use a back-up pack for electrical medical equipment, such as an IV pump. Back-up packs do not last more than 24 hours, so call emergency services.

Hurricanes

G Know what category the hurricane is and track the expected path.

G Know which clients must go to shelters, skilled nursing facilities, hospitals, or other facilities, and which need special assistance. Be aware of people with special needs. High-risk people include the elderly and those unable to evacuate on their own. High-risk areas include mobile homes or trailers.

G Call your employer for instructions.

G Contact your clients if instructed to do so.

G Fill the bathtub with fresh water.

G Board up windows.

G Evacuate if advised to do so.

G Check the fuel level in automobiles.

G Have a portable battery-operated radio, flashlight, and cooking equipment available.

G Be aware of people with special needs.

Earthquakes

If indoors, follow these guidelines:

G Drop to the ground.

G If possible, get under a sturdy piece of furniture, such as a heavy table, and hold on until the shaking stops.

G If no table or desk is available, stay crouched down in the inside corner of a building or house, and cover your face and head with your arms.

G Stay away from windows, outside walls, and anything that might fall over or fall down.

G Do not exit a building or house during the shaking.

G Do not use elevators.

If outdoors, follow these guidelines:

G Move away from buildings, electric poles and wires, and streetlights. Falling or flying debris is a far greater danger than ground movement.

G If driving, stop as quickly as is safely possible and stay in the vehicle. Avoid stopping under overpasses or near buildings or wires if possible.

G If trapped under debris after an earthquake, do not light a match or ignite a lighter, and avoid kicking up dust. Breathe through a handkerchief or clothing and make tapping noises or use a whistle, if available, to get rescuers' attention. Do not shout. Shouting could cause you to inhale dangerous amounts of dust.

III. Understanding Clients

Culture and Family

Basic Human Needs

People have different genes, physical appearances, cultural backgrounds, ages, and social or financial positions. But all human beings have the same basic physical needs:

- Food and water
- Protection and shelter
- Activity
- Sleep and rest
- Comfort, especially freedom from pain

People also have **psychosocial needs**, which involve social interaction, emotions, intellect, and spirituality. Although they are not as easy to define as physical needs, psychosocial needs include the following:

- Love and affection
- Acceptance by others
- Safety and security
- Self-reliance and independence in daily living
- Contact with others
- Success and self-esteem

Health and well-being affect how well psychosocial needs are met. Stress and frustration occur when basic needs are not met. This can lead to fear, anxiety, anger, aggression, withdrawal, indifference, and depression. Stress can also cause physical problems that may eventually lead to illness.

Abraham Maslow was a researcher of human behavior. He wrote about human physical and psychosocial needs. He arranged these needs by order of importance. He thought that physical needs must be met before psychosocial needs can be met. His theory is called *Maslow's Hierarchy of Needs* (Fig. 3-1).

Humans are sexual beings. They continue to have sexual needs throughout their lives. Sexual urges do not end due to age. Clients have the right to choose how they express their sexuality. In all age groups, there is a variety of sexual behavior. This is also true of clients.

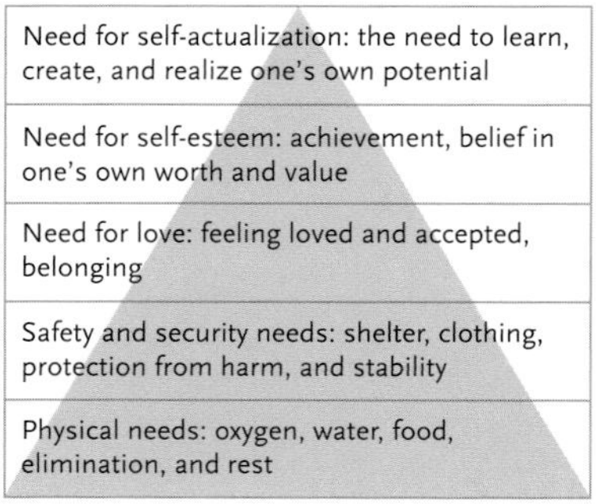

Need for self-actualization: the need to learn, create, and realize one's own potential
Need for self-esteem: achievement, belief in one's own worth and value
Need for love: feeling loved and accepted, belonging
Safety and security needs: shelter, clothing, protection from harm, and stability
Physical needs: oxygen, water, food, elimination, and rest

It is important that HHAs always knock or announce themselves before entering clients' rooms. They should listen and wait for a response before entering. If an HHA encounters a sexual situation between consenting adults, he should provide privacy and leave the room.

Fig. 3-1. *Maslow's Hierarchy of Needs is a model developed by Abraham Maslow to show how physical and psychosocial needs are arranged in order of importance.*

HHAs should be open and nonjudgmental about clients' sexual attitudes. They must respect clients' sexual orientation. No matter what an HHA's personal or religious feelings regarding sexuality may be, he should always treat clients with respect.

Cultural Differences

People come from many different cultural backgrounds and traditions. HHAs will take care of clients with backgrounds and traditions different from their own. It is important that HHAs respect and value each person as an individual. They should respond to differences and new experiences with acceptance.

There are so many different cultures that they cannot all be listed here. A **culture** is a system of learned behaviors, practiced by a group of people, that are considered to be the tradition of that group and are passed on from one generation to the next. Each culture may have different knowledge, behaviors, beliefs, values, attitudes, religions, and customs. One might talk about American culture being different from Japanese culture. But within American culture there are thousands of different groups with their own cultures. Japanese Americans, African Americans, and Native Americans are just a few. Even people from a particular region, state, or city can be said to have a different culture. The culture of the South is not the same as the culture of New York City.

Cultural background affects how friendly people are to strangers. It can affect how they feel about having people in their homes, or how close they want others to stand to them when talking. It can affect how they feel about HHAs performing care for them or discussing their health with them. HHAs should be sensitive to clients' backgrounds and preferences. They may have to adjust their behavior around some clients. Regardless of background, all clients must be treated with respect and professionalism. HHAs should expect to be treated respectfully as well.

Religious differences also influence the way people behave. Religion can be very important in people's lives, particularly when they are ill or dying. HHAs must respect clients' religious beliefs and practices, even if they are different from their own. They should not question clients' beliefs or discuss their beliefs with clients.

In addition to showing respect for different cultural and religious traditions, there may be specific practices that affect an HHA's work. Many religious beliefs include dietary restrictions. These are rules about what and when followers can eat and drink. For example, many Jewish people do not eat pork. The HHA should check with his agency if he is unsure about planning and preparing meals for clients. Any dietary restrictions should be honored.

Some people's backgrounds may make them less comfortable being touched. An HHA should ask permission before touching clients. He should be sensitive to their feelings. HHAs must touch clients in order to do their jobs. However, they should recognize that some clients feel more comfortable when there is little physical contact.

Person-Directed (Person-Centered) Care

Some long-term care facilities and other healthcare settings have adopted models of care that promote meaningful environments with individualized approaches to care. Person-directed care emphasizes the individuality of the person who needs care. Core values are promoting choice, dignity, respect, self-determination, and purposeful living. The Pioneer Network and The Eden Alternative are organizations concerned with promoting person-directed care. Their websites, pioneernetwork.net and edenalt.org, have more information.

Families

Families play an important part in most people's lives. There are many different kinds of families:

- Nuclear families (two parents and one or more children)
- Single-parent families (one parent and one or more children)

- Married or committed couples of the same sex or opposite sex, with or without children
- Extended families (parents, children, grandparents, aunts, uncles, cousins, other relatives, and even friends)
- Blended families (divorced or widowed parents who have remarried and have children from previous relationships and/or the current marriage)

Family members help in many ways:

- Helping clients make care decisions
- Communicating with the care team
- Providing daily care when home health aide is not present
- Giving support and encouragement
- Connecting the client to the outside world
- Offering assurance to dying clients that family memories and traditions will be valued and carried on

Body Systems

Each system in the body has a condition under which it works best. **Homeostasis** is the name for the condition in which all of the body's systems are working at their best. To be in homeostasis, the body's **metabolism**, or physical and chemical processes, must be working at a steady level. When disease or injury occurs, the body's metabolism is disturbed. Homeostasis is lost. Changes in metabolic processes are called signs and symptoms. Noticing and reporting changes in clients is a very important part of an HHA's job. Changes could be signs of problems.

Each system in the body has its own unique structure and function. Body systems can be broken down in different ways. In this book the human body is divided into ten systems:

1. Integumentary (skin)
2. Musculoskeletal
3. Nervous
4. Circulatory or Cardiovascular
5. Respiratory
6. Urinary
7. Gastrointestinal
8. Endocrine
9. Reproductive
10. Immune and Lymphatic

Body systems are made up of organs. An organ has a specific function. Organs are made up of tissues. Tissues are made up of groups of cells that perform a similar task. For example, the heart is one of the organs in the circulatory system. It is made up of tissues and cells. Cells are the building blocks of the body. Living cells divide, grow, and die, renewing the tissues and organs of the body.

Common Disorders/Observing and Reporting

1. The Integumentary System

The largest organ and system in the body is the skin. Skin is a natural protective covering, or integument. Skin prevents injury to internal organs. It also protects the body against entry of bacteria. Skin also prevents the loss of too much water, which is essential to life. Skin is made up of layers of tissue. Within these layers are sweat glands, which secrete sweat to help cool the body when needed, and sebaceous glands, which secrete oil (sebum) to keep the skin lubricated. There are also hair follicles, many tiny blood vessels (capillaries), and tiny nerve endings.

The skin is also a sense organ. It feels heat, cold, pain, touch, and pressure. It then tells the brain what it is feeling. Body temperature is regulated in the skin. Blood vessels **dilate**, or widen, when the outside temperature is too high. This brings more blood to the body surface to cool it off. The same blood vessels **constrict**, or narrow, when the outside temperature is too cold. By restricting the amount of blood reaching the skin, the blood vessels help the body retain heat.

Common Disorders: Integumentary System

C/D Pressure ulcers, or decubitus ulcers

C/D **Shingles**

C/D **Scabies**

C/D Wounds

C/D Fungal infections

C/D Dermatitis (inflammation of the skin)

Observing and Reporting: Integumentary System

O/R Pale, white, reddened, or purple areas

O/R Blisters or bruises

O/R Complaints of tingling, warmth, or burning

O/R Dry or flaking skin

O/R Rashes or any skin discoloration

O/R Swelling

O/R Cuts, boils, wounds, abrasions

O/R Fluid or blood draining from the skin

O/R Broken skin

O/R Changes in moistness/dryness

O/R Changes in wound or ulcer (size, depth, drainage, color, odor)

O/R Redness or broken skin between toes or around toenails

O/R Scalp or hair changes

O/R Skin that appears different from normal or that has changed

O/R In darker complexions, any change in the feel of the tissue; any change in the appearance of the skin, such as an "orange-peel" look or a purplish hue; and extremely dry, crust-like areas that might be covering a tissue break

2. The Musculoskeletal System

Muscles, bones, ligaments, tendons, and cartilage give the body shape and structure. They work together to move the body. Besides allowing the body to move, bones also protect organs. Muscles are connected to bone by tendons. Muscles provide movement of body parts to maintain posture and to produce heat. Exercise is important for improving and maintaining physical and mental health. Inactivity and immobility can result in a loss of self-esteem, depression, pneumonia, and urinary tract infections. They can also lead to constipation, blood clots, dulling of the senses, and muscle **atrophy** or **contractures**. Range of motion (ROM) exercises can help prevent these conditions.

Common Disorders: Musculoskeletal System

C/D **Fractures**

C/D **Osteoporosis**

C/D Arthritis

Observing and Reporting: Musculoskeletal System

O/R Changes in ability to perform routine movements and activities

O/R Any changes in client's ability to perform ROM exercises

O/R Pain during movement

O/R Any new or increased swelling of joints

O/R White, shiny, red, or warm areas over a joint

O/R Bruising

O/R Aches and pains reported

3. The Nervous System

The nervous system is the control and message center of the body. It controls and coordinates all body functions. The nervous system also senses and interprets information from outside the human body.

Common Disorders: Central Nervous System

C/D **Dementia**, including Alzheimer's disease

C/D Cerebrovascular accident (CVA), or stroke

C/D Parkinson's disease

C/D **Multiple sclerosis**

C/D **Epilepsy**

C/D Cerebral palsy

C/D Head and spinal cord injuries

Observing and Reporting: Central Nervous System

O/R Fatigue or pain with movement or exercise

O/R Shaking or trembling

O/R Inability to move one side of body

O/R Difficulty speaking or slurring of speech

O/R Numbness or tingling

O/R Disturbance or changes in vision or hearing

O/R Dizziness or loss of balance

O/R Changes in eating patterns and/or fluid intake

O/R Difficulty swallowing

O/R Bowel and bladder changes

O/R Depression or mood changes

O/R Memory loss or confusion

O/R Violent behavior

O/R Any unusual or unexplained change in behavior

O/R Decreased ability to perform ADLs

The Nervous System: Sense Organs

The eyes, ears, nose, tongue, and skin are the body's major sense organs. They are part of the central nervous system because they receive impulses from the environment. They relay these impulses to the nerves.

Common Disorders: Eyes and Ears

c/D   Cataracts

c/D   **Glaucoma**

c/D   **Age-related macular degeneration** (**AMD**)

c/D   Otitis media (infection of the middle ear)

c/D   Deafness

c/D   Vertigo (dizziness)

Observing and Reporting: Eyes and Ears

O/R   Changes in vision or hearing

O/R   Signs of infection

O/R   Dizziness

O/R   Complaints of pain in eyes or ears

4. The Circulatory or Cardiovascular System

The circulatory system is made up of the heart, blood vessels, and blood. The heart pumps blood through the blood vessels to the cells. The blood carries food, oxygen, and other substances that cells need to function properly.

The circulatory system supplies food, oxygen, and hormones to cells. It supplies the body with infection-fighting blood cells. The circulatory system removes waste products from cells and also helps control body temperature.

Common Disorders: Circulatory System

c/D   Atherosclerosis (hardening and narrowing of the blood vessels)

c/D   Myocardial infarction (MI), or heart attack

c/D   Angina pectoris (chest pain, pressure, or discomfort)

c/D   Hypertension, or high blood pressure

c/D   Congestive heart failure (heart is no longer able to pump effectively)

c/D   Peripheral vascular disease (poor circulation to extremities)

Observing and Reporting: Circulatory System

O/R   Changes in pulse rate

O/R   Weakness, fatigue

O/R   Loss of ability to perform activities of daily living (ADLs)

O/R   Swelling of ankles, feet, fingers, or hands (edema)

O/R   Pale or bluish hands, feet, or lips

O/R   Chest pain

O/R   Weight gain

O/R   Shortness of breath, changes in breathing patterns, or inability to catch breath

O/R   Severe headache

O/R   Inactivity (which can lead to circulatory problems)

5. The Respiratory System

Respiration, the body taking in oxygen and removing carbon dioxide, involves breathing in (inspiration), and breathing out (expiration). The lungs accomplish this process. The functions of the respiratory system are to bring oxygen into the body and to eliminate carbon dioxide produced as the body uses oxygen.

Common Disorders: Respiratory System

C/D   **Asthma**

C/D   Upper respiratory infection (URI), or a cold

C/D   **Chronic obstructive pulmonary disease (COPD)**

C/D   **Bronchitis**

C/D   Pneumonia

C/D   Emphysema

C/D   Lung cancer

C/D   **Tuberculosis**

Observing and Reporting: Respiratory System

O/R   Change in respiratory rate

O/R   Shallow breathing or breathing through pursed lips

O/R   Coughing or wheezing

O/R   Nasal congestion or discharge

O/R   Sore throat, difficulty swallowing, or swollen tonsils

O/R The need to sit after mild exertion

O/R Pale, bluish, or gray color of the lips, arms, and/or legs (cyanosis)

O/R Pain in the chest area

O/R Discolored **sputum** (green, yellow, blood-tinged, or gray)

6. The Urinary System

The urinary system is composed of two kidneys, two ureters, one urinary bladder, a single urethra, and a meatus. The urinary system has two important functions. Through urine, the urinary system eliminates waste products created by the cells. The urinary system also maintains the water balance in the body.

Common Disorders: Urinary System

C/D Urinary incontinence

C/D Urinary tract infection (UTI), or cystitis

C/D Calculi (kidney stones)

C/D Nephritis (inflammation of the kidneys)

C/D Renovascular hypertension

C/D Chronic renal failure (CRF), or chronic kidney failure

Observing and Reporting: Urinary System

O/R Weight loss or gain

O/R Swelling in the upper or lower extremities

O/R Pain or burning during urination (dysuria)

O/R Changes in urine, such as cloudiness, odor, or color

O/R Changes in frequency and amount of urination

O/R Swelling in the abdominal/bladder area

O/R Complaints that bladder feels full or painful

O/R Urinary incontinence/dribbling

O/R Pain in the kidney or back/flank region

O/R Inadequate fluid intake

7. The Gastrointestinal (GI) System

The gastrointestinal (GI) system, also called the digestive system, is made up of the gastrointestinal tract and the accessory digestive organs. The gastrointestinal system has two functions: **digestion** and **elimination**.

Common Disorders: Gastrointestinal System

C/D Heartburn

C/D **Gastroesophageal reflux disease (GERD)**

C/D Peptic ulcers

C/D **Constipation**

C/D **Diarrhea**

C/D **Hepatitis**

C/D Ulcerative colitis

C/D Colitis

C/D Colorectal cancer

C/D Hemorrhoids

C/D Diverticulitis

Observing and Reporting: Gastrointestinal System

O/R Difficulty swallowing or chewing (including denture problems, tooth pain, or mouth sores)

O/R Fecal incontinence (inability to control the bowels, leading to involuntary passage of stool)

O/R Weight gain or weight loss

O/R Loss of appetite

O/R Abdominal pain and cramping

O/R Diarrhea

O/R Nausea and vomiting (especially vomitus that looks like coffee grounds)

O/R Constipation

O/R Flatulence/gas

O/R Hiccups, belching

O/R Bloody, black, or hard stools

O/R Heartburn

O/R Poor nutritional intake

8. The Endocrine System

The endocrine system is made up of glands in different areas of the body. **Glands** are organs that produce and secrete chemicals called hormones.

Hormones are chemical substances created by the body that control numerous body functions. The functions of the endocrine system are to

- Maintain homeostasis
- Influence growth and development
- Regulate levels of sugar in the blood
- Regulate levels of calcium in the bones
- Regulate the body's ability to reproduce
- Determine how fast cells burn food for energy

Common Disorders: Endocrine System

C/D Diabetes

C/D Hyperthyroidism

C/D Hypothyroidism

Observing and Reporting: Endocrine System

O/R Headache

O/R Weakness

O/R Blurred vision

O/R Dizziness

O/R Irritability

O/R Sweating/excessive perspiration

O/R Change in "normal" behavior

O/R Confusion

O/R Change in mobility

O/R Change in sensation

O/R Numbness or tingling in arms or legs

O/R Weight gain or weight loss

O/R Loss of appetite or increased appetite

O/R Increased thirst

O/R Frequent urination or any change in urine output

O/R Hunger

O/R Dry skin

O/R Skin breakdown

O/R Sweet or fruity breath

^O/_R Sluggishness or fatigue

^O/_R Hyperactivity

9. The Reproductive System

The reproductive system is made up of the reproductive organs, which are different in men and women. The reproductive system allows human beings to reproduce, or create new human life. Reproduction begins when a male's and female's sex cells (sperm and ovum) join. These sex cells are formed in the male and female sex glands, called the *gonads*.

Common Disorders: Reproductive System

^C/_D Vaginitis

^C/_D Benign prostatic hypertrophy (BPH) (enlarged prostate causes problems with urination)

^C/_D **Sexually transmitted infections (STIs)** (chlamydia, syphilis, gonorrhea, genital herpes)

Observing and Reporting: Reproductive System

^O/_R Discomfort or difficulty with urination

^O/_R Discharge from the penis or vagina

^O/_R Swelling of the genitals

^O/_R Blood in urine or stool

^O/_R Breast changes, including size, shape, lumps, or discharge from the nipple

^O/_R Sores on the genitals

^O/_R Redness, rash on genitals

^O/_R Genital itching

^O/_R Client reports of erectile dysfunction (ED), or trouble getting or keeping an erection

^O/_R Client reports of painful intercourse

10. The Immune and Lymphatic Systems

The immune system protects the body from disease-causing bacteria, viruses, and organisms in two ways. Nonspecific immunity protects the body from disease in general. Specific immunity protects against a particular disease that is invading the body at a given time.

The lymphatic system removes excess fluids and waste products from the body's tissues. It also helps the immune system fight infection. The lymphatic system consists of lymph vessels and lymph capillaries in which a fluid called lymph circulates.

Common Disorders: Immune and Lymphatic Systems

C/D **HIV** and **AIDS**

C/D Lymphoma

Observing and Reporting: Immune and Lymphatic Systems

O/R Recurring infections (such as fevers and diarrhea)

O/R Swelling of the lymph nodes

O/R Increased fatigue

Human Development

Stages/Common Disorders

Throughout their lives, people change physically and psychologically. Everyone will go through the same stages of development. However, no two people will follow the exact pattern or rate of development. Each client must be treated as an individual and as a whole person who is growing and developing, rather than someone who is merely ill or disabled.

Infancy (Birth to 12 Months)

Infants grow and develop very quickly. In one year a baby moves from total dependence to the relative independence of moving around, communicating basic needs, and feeding himself. Physical development in infancy moves from the head down. For example, infants gain control over the muscles of the neck before the muscles in their shoulders. Control over muscles in the trunk area, such as the shoulders, develops before control of the arms and legs. This head-to-toe sequence should be respected when caring for infants. For example, newborns must be supported at the shoulders, head, and neck. Babies who cannot sit or crawl should not be encouraged to stand or walk.

Common Disorders: Infancy

C/D Prematurity

C/D Low birth weight

C/D Birth defects (cerebral palsy, cystic fibrosis, Down syndrome) c/ᴅ   Viral or bacterial infections

c/ᴅ   Sudden infant death syndrome (SIDS)

Toddler (Ages 1 to 3)

During the toddler years, children gain independence. One part of this independence is new control over their bodies. Toddlers learn to speak, gain coordination of their limbs, and learn to control their bladders and bowels. Toddlers assert their new independence by exploring. Poisons and other hazards, such as sharp objects, must be locked away. Psychologically, toddlers learn that they are individuals, separate from their parents. Children of this age may try to control their parents. They may try to get what they want by throwing tantrums, whining, or refusing to cooperate. This is a key time for parents to set rules and standards.

Preschool (Ages 3 to 6)

Children in their preschool years develop skills that will help them become more independent and have social relationships. They develop vocabulary and language skills. They learn to play in groups. They become more physically coordinated and learn to care for themselves. Preschoolers also develop ways of relating to family members. They begin to learn right from wrong.

School-Age (Ages 6 to 10)

From ages 6 to about 10 years, children's development is centered on **cognitive** (related to thinking and learning skills) and social development. As children enter school, they also explore the world around them. They relate to other children through games, peer groups, and classroom activities. In these years, children learn to get along with each other. They also begin to behave in ways common to their gender. They begin to develop a conscience, morals, and self-esteem.

Common Disorders: Childhood

c/ᴅ   Chickenpox

c/ᴅ   Viral or bacterial infections

c/ᴅ   Leukemia

c/ᴅ   Child abuse

Preadolescence (Ages 10 to 13)

During the years between 10 and 13, children enjoy a growing sense of self-identity and a strong sense of identity with their peers. They tend to be very social. This is usually a relatively calm period, and preadolescents are often easy to get along with and able to handle more responsibility at home and school. Childhood fears of ghosts or monsters will give way to fears based in the real world. It is important that preadolescents feel able to trust in the attention and care of parents or other adults.

Adolescence (Ages 13 to 19)

The start of puberty marks the beginning of adolescence. Puberty is the stage of growth when secondary sex characteristics, such as body hair, appear. Reproductive organs begin to function. The body begins to secrete reproductive hormones. Although it varies, puberty generally occurs between the ages of 10 and 14 for girls and 12 and 16 for boys.

Many teenagers have a hard time adapting to the changes that occur in their bodies during puberty. Peer acceptance is important to them. Adolescents may be afraid that they are unattractive or abnormal. This concern for body image and acceptance, combined with changing hormones that influence emotions, can cause rapid mood swings. Pressures develop as they remain dependent on their parents and yet need to express themselves socially and sexually. This causes conflict and stress.

Common Disorders: Adolescence

- C/D   Eating disorders (**anorexia**, bulimia)
- C/D   Sexually-transmitted infections (STIs)
- C/D   Teenage pregnancy
- C/D   Depression
- C/D   Trauma or accidental injury

Young Adulthood (Ages 19 to 40)

Physical growth has usually been completed by this time. Adopting a healthy lifestyle in these years can make life better now and prevent health problems in later adulthood. Psychological and social development continues, however. The developmental tasks of these years include choosing an appropriate education and an occupation or career, selecting a mate, learning to live with a mate or others, raising children, and developing a satisfying sex life.

Middle Adulthood (Ages 40 to 65)

In general, people in middle adulthood are more comfortable and stable than they were before. Many of their major life decisions have already been made. Physical changes related to aging also occur in middle adulthood. Adults in this age group may notice that they have difficulty maintaining their weight or notice a decrease in strength and energy. Metabolism and other body functions slow down. Wrinkles and gray hair appear. Many diseases and illnesses can develop in these years. These disorders can become chronic and life-threatening.

Late Adulthood (65 Years and Older)

Persons in late adulthood must adjust to the effects of aging. These changes can include the loss of strength and health, the death of loved ones, retirement, and preparation for their own death. The developmental tasks of this age seem to deal entirely with loss. But solutions to these problems often involve new relationships, friendships, and interests.

Common disorders for this age group are discussed in Section V.

Aging

Aging causes many changes. However, normal changes of aging do not mean an older person must become dependent, ill, or inactive. Knowing how to tell normal changes of aging from signs of illness or disability will allow HHAs to better help clients. Normal changes of aging include the following:

- Skin is thinner, drier, more fragile, and less elastic.
- Muscles weaken and lose tone.
- Bones lose density and become more brittle.
- Sensitivity of nerve endings in the skin decreases.
- Responses and reflexes slow.
- Short-term memory loss occurs.
- Senses of vision, hearing, taste, touch, and smell weaken.
- Heart works less efficiently.
- Oxygen in the blood decreases.
- Appetite decreases.
- Urinary elimination is more frequent.
- Digestion takes longer and is less efficient.
- Levels of hormones decrease.
- Immunity weakens.
- Lifestyle changes occur.

There are also changes that are NOT considered normal changes of aging and should be reported to the supervisor, including the following:

- Signs of depression
- Suicidal thoughts
- Loss of ability to think logically
- Disorientation
- Confusion
- Poor nutrition
- Shortness of breath
- Incontinence

This is not a complete list. The HHA's job includes reporting any change, normal or not.

Death

Death can occur suddenly without warning, or it can be expected. Older people or those with terminal illnesses may have time to prepare for death. A **terminal illness** is a disease or condition that will eventually cause death. Preparing for death is a process that affects the dying person's emotions and behavior.

Dr. Elisabeth Kübler-Ross studied and wrote about the grief process. Her book, *On Death and Dying*, describes five stages that dying people and their loved ones may reach before death. Not all people go through all the stages. These five stages are listed below.

- **Denial**: People in the denial stage may refuse to believe they are dying. They often believe a mistake has been made.
- **Anger**: Once they start to face the possibility of their death, people may become angry that they are dying.
- **Bargaining**: Once people have begun to believe that they are dying, they may make promises to God, care providers, or others. They may somehow try to bargain for their recovery.
- **Depression**: As dying people become weaker and symptoms get worse, they may become deeply sad or depressed.
- **Acceptance**: Many people who are dying are eventually able to accept death and prepare for it. They may make plans for their last days or for the ceremonies that may follow their death.

Death is a very sensitive topic. Many people find it hard to discuss death. Feelings and attitudes about death can be formed by many factors:

- Experience with death

- Personality type
- Religious beliefs
- Cultural background

Guidelines: Caring for the Dying Client

G   **Diminished senses**: Reduce glare and keep room lighting low. Hearing is usually the last sense to leave the body. Speak in a normal tone. Tell the person about any procedures that are being done and what is happening in the room. Do not expect an answer. Ask few questions. Observe body language to anticipate client's needs.

G   **Care of the mouth and nose**: Give mouth care often. If the client is unconscious, give mouth care every two hours. Apply lubricant, such as lip balm, to the lips and nose.

G   **Skin care**: Give bed baths and incontinence care as needed. Bathe perspiring clients often. Skin should be kept clean and dry. Change sheets and clothes for comfort. Keep sheets wrinkle-free. Skin care to prevent pressure ulcers is important.

G   **Comfort**: Pain relief is critical. Observe for signs of pain and report them. Frequent changes of position, back massage, skin care, mouth care, and proper body alignment may help.

G   **Environment**: Put favorite objects and photographs where the client can easily see them. Make sure room is comfortable, appropriately lit, and well-ventilated.

G   **Emotional and spiritual support**: Listening may be one of the most important things you can do for a dying client. Listen if the client wishes to talk. Touch can be important. Do not avoid the dying person or his family. Do not deny that death is approaching. Do not tell the client that anyone knows how or when it will happen. Some clients may seek spiritual comfort from clergy. Give privacy for visits from clergy, family, and friends. Do not discuss your religious or spiritual beliefs with clients or their families or make recommendations.

HHAs can treat clients with dignity when they are approaching death by respecting their rights and their preferences. There are some legal rights to remember when caring for people who are dying:

- The right to refuse treatment
- The right to have visitors
- The right to privacy

Common signs of approaching death include the following:

- Blurred and failing vision
- Unfocused eyes
- Impaired speech
- Diminished sense of touch
- Loss of movement, muscle tone, and feeling
- A rising or below-normal body temperature
- Decreasing blood pressure
- Weak pulse that is abnormally slow or rapid
- Alternating slow, irregular respirations and rapid, shallow respirations
- A rattling or gurgling sound as the person breathes
- Cold, pale skin
- Mottling (bruised appearance), spotting, or blotching of skin caused by poor circulation
- Perspiration
- Incontinence (both urine and stool)
- Disorientation or confusion

Postmortem care is care of the body after death. It takes place after the client has been declared dead by a nurse or doctor. HHAs must be sensitive to the needs of the family and friends after clients have died. They should follow their agency's policies and only perform assigned tasks.

Guidelines: Postmortem Care

G   Bathe the body. Be gentle to avoid bruising. Place drainage pads where needed. Follow Standard Precautions.

G   Check with family about how to dress client and whether or not to remove jewelry.

G   Do not remove any tubes or other equipment.

G   If instructed, put dentures back in the mouth and close the mouth.

G   Close the eyes carefully.

G   Position the body on the back with legs straight and arms folded across the abdomen. Place a small pillow under the head.

G   Strip the bed after body has been removed.

G   Open windows to air room as needed and straighten up.

G   Arrange personal items carefully so they are not lost.

G   Document according to your agency's policy.

Dealing with grief after the death of a loved one is an individual process. No two people will grieve in exactly the same way. It is also a changing or adaptive process. Feelings may change from day to day, or even hour to hour. This is normal. Clergy, counselors, or social workers can provide help for people who are grieving. Family members or friends may have any of these reactions to the death of a loved one:

- Shock

- Denial

- Anger

- Guilt

- Regret

- Relief

- Sadness

- Loneliness

Hospice Care

Hospice care is the term for the special care that a dying person needs. It is a compassionate way to care for dying people and their families. Hospice care uses a holistic approach. It treats the person's physical, emotional, spiritual, and social needs. Hospice care can be given seven days a week, 24 hours a day. Hospice care may be given in a hospital, at a care facility, or in the home. A hospice can be any location where a person who is dying is treated with dignity by caregivers. Any caregiver may give hospice care, but often specially-trained nurses and volunteers provide it.

Hospice care helps to meet all needs of the dying person. The client, her family, and her friends are directly involved in care decisions. The client is encouraged to participate in family life and decision-making as long as possible.

In home care, goals usually focus on recovery, or on the client's ability to care for herself as much as possible. In hospice care, however, the goals of care are the comfort and dignity of the client. This is an important difference. HHAs will need to change their focus when caring for hospice clients. The focus should be on pain relief and comfort, rather than on teaching clients to care for themselves.

Clients who are dying need to feel independent for as long as possible. Caregivers should allow clients to retain as much control over their lives as possible. Eventually, caregivers may have to meet all of the client's basic needs.

Family members or friends who are caregivers for the dying person will appreciate help from HHAs. HHAs are providing them with a break. This kind of care is sometimes referred to as *respite care*. Family caregivers should be encouraged to take breaks and take care of themselves. However, an HHA should not insist that they do so. Many want to do all they can for their loved one during his or her last days. The HHA should observe family caregivers for signs of excessive stress and report them to the supervisor. The home health agency may be able to refer them to local support services.

Guidelines: Hospice Care

G   Be a good listener, but do not push a client or family member to talk.

G   Respect privacy and independence.

G   Be sensitive to individual needs. Ask how you can be of help.

G   Be aware of your own feelings. Know your limits and respect them.

G   Follow the plan of care.

G   Take good care of yourself.

G   Allow yourself to grieve. You will develop close relationships with some clients. Know that it is normal to feel sad, angry, or lonely when clients die.

IV. Client Care

Maintaining Mobility, Skin, and Comfort

Positioning

Clients who spend a lot of time in bed often need help getting into comfortable positions. They also need to change positions periodically to avoid muscle stiffness and skin breakdown or pressure ulcers. Bed-bound clients should be repositioned at least every two hours. Each time there is a change, the HHA should document the position and the time. Following are the five basic body positions:

1. Supine, or lying flat on back (Fig. 4-1)

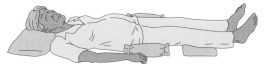

Fig. 4-1. *A person in the supine position is lying flat on his or her back.*

2. Lateral, or lying on either side (Fig. 4-2)

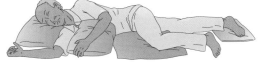

Fig. 4-2. *A person in the lateral position is lying on his or her side.*

3. Prone, or lying on the stomach (Fig. 4-3)

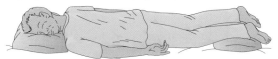

Fig. 4-3. *A person in the prone position is lying on his or her stomach.*

4. Fowler's, or semi-sitting position (45 to 60 degrees) (Fig. 4-4)

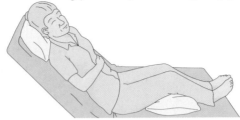

Fig. 4-4. *A person lying in the Fowler's position is partially reclined.*

5. Sims', or lying on the left side with one leg drawn up (Fig. 4-5)

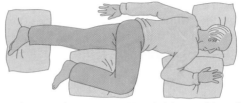

Fig. 4-5. *A person lying in the Sims' position is lying on his or her left side with one leg drawn up.*

Clients who are confined to bed need to maintain proper body alignment. This promotes recovery and prevents injury to muscles and joints. These guidelines help clients maintain proper alignment and make progress when they can get out of bed:

Guidelines: Alignment and Positioning

G   Observe principles of alignment. Proper alignment is based on straight lines. The spine should be in a straight line. Pillows or rolled or folded blankets can support the small of the back and raise the knees or head in the supine position. They can support the head and one leg in the lateral position.

G   Keep body parts in natural positions. In a natural hand position, the fingers are slightly curled. Use a rolled washcloth, gauze bandage, or a rubber ball inside the palm to support the fingers in this position. Use bed cradles to keep covers from resting on feet in the supine position.

G   Prevent external rotation of hips. When legs and hips turn outward during bed rest, hip contractures can result. A rolled blanket or towel that is tucked alongside the hip and thigh can keep the leg from turning outward.

G   Change positions often to prevent muscle stiffness and pressure ulcers. This should be done at least every two hours. The position used depends on the client's condition and preference. Check the skin every time you reposition a client.

G Have plenty of pillows available to provide support in the various positions.

G Use positioning devices (backrests, bed cradles, **draw sheets**, foot-boards, and handrolls).

G Splints may be prescribed by a doctor to keep a client's joints in the correct position.

G Give back rubs for comfort and relaxation.

The *Comfort Measures* material later in this section contains more information on using positioning devices for comfort.

HHAs must remember to use proper body mechanics when moving or positioning a client. Lifting should be avoided whenever possible. Pushing, rolling, sliding, or pivoting is much safer.

Before a client who has been lying down stands up, he should dangle. To **dangle** means to sit up on the side of the bed with the legs hanging over the side. This helps clients regain balance before standing up and allows blood pressure to stabilize. For some clients who are unable to walk, sitting up and dangling the legs for a few minutes may be ordered.

Assisting a client to sit up on side of bed: dangling

1. Wash your hands.

2. Explain the procedure to the client, speaking clearly, slowly, and directly. Maintain face-to-face contact whenever possible.

3. Provide privacy if the client desires it.

4. If the bed is adjustable, adjust bed to lowest position. If the bed is movable, lock bed wheels.

5. Raise the head of the bed to a sitting position. Fanfold (fold into pleats) the top covers to the foot of the bed.

6. Stand with feet shoulder-width apart. Bend your knees.

7. Place one arm under the client's shoulder blades. Place the

other arm under the client's thighs (Fig. 4-6).

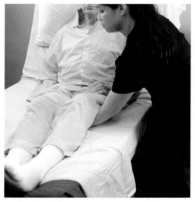

Fig. 4-6. One arm should be under the client's shoulder blades and the other arm should be under the thighs.

8. On the count of three, slowly turn client into a sitting position with legs dangling over the side of the bed (Fig. 4-7).

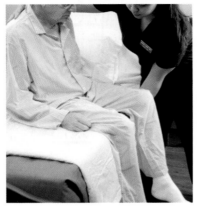

Fig. 4-7. *The weight of the client's legs hanging down from the bed helps the client sit up.*

9. Ask client to hold on to edge of mattress with both hands. Put nonskid shoes on the client.

10. Have client dangle as long as ordered. The care plan may direct you to allow the client to dangle for several minutes and then return him to lying down, or it may direct you to allow the client to dangle in preparation for walking or a transfer. Follow the care plan. Do not leave the client alone. If the client is dizzy for more than a minute, have him lie down again. Take his pulse and respiration rates and report to your supervisor.

11. Remove client's shoes.

12. Gently assist client back into bed. Place one arm around client's shoulders. Place the other arm under client's knees. Slowly swing client's legs onto bed.

13. Leave bed in lowest position.

14. Wash your hands.

15. Document the procedure and your observations. How did the client tolerate sitting up? Did the client become dizzy?

Transfers and Ambulation

Transferring a client means that the HHA is moving him from one place to another. Transfers can move a client from a wheelchair to a bed, from a bed to a chair, and so on.

Safety is one of the most important things to consider during transfers. A **transfer belt** is a safety device used to transfer clients who are weak, unsteady, or uncoordinated. It is called a **gait belt** when it is used to help clients walk. The belt is made of canvas or other heavy material. It has a buckle and sometimes has handles. It fits around the client's waist outside the clothing. It should never be placed on bare skin. The belt gives caregivers something firm to hold on to when helping with transfers. When applying a transfer belt, the HHA should place the belt over the client's clothing and around the waist. She should tighten the buckle until it is snug, leaving enough room to insert flat fingers comfortably under the belt. The HHA should make sure that skin or skin folds (for example, breasts) are not caught under the belt.

Guidelines: Wheelchairs

G   Learn how each wheelchair works. Know how to apply and release the brake and how to operate the armrests and footrests. Always lock the wheelchair before helping a client into or out of it. After a transfer, unlock the wheelchair.

G   To transfer to or from a wheelchair, the client must use the side of the body that can bear weight to support and lift the side that cannot bear weight.

G   Before any transfer, make sure the client is wearing nonskid footwear that is securely fastened. This promotes the client's safety and reduces the risk of falls.

G   Make sure the client is safe and comfortable during transfers. Ask the client how you can help. Some clients may only want you to bring the chair to the bedside. Others may want you to be more involved.

G   Keep the client's body in proper alignment while in a wheelchair or chair. Special cushions and pillows can be used for support. The hips should be well-positioned back in the chair.

G   When a client is in a wheelchair or any chair, he or she should be repositioned at least every hour.

Falls

If a client starts to fall during a transfer, the HHA should do the following:

- Widen his stance.

- Bring the client's body close to him to break the fall.

- Bend his knees and support the client as he lowers the client to the floor. The HHA may need to drop to the floor with the client to avoid injury to himself or the client.

The HHA should not try to reverse or stop a fall. He or the client can suffer worse injuries if he tries to stop, rather than break, a fall. If a client has fallen, the HHA should call for help if a family member is around. He should not try to get the client up after the fall unless he is certain the client is not injured. Many agencies do not allow staff to help a client up after a fall until the client has been evaluated by a nurse. The HHA should always call his supervisor if he is unsure of what to do. If he does help the client up, he should get her in bed, take her vital signs, then report the fall to his supervisor immediately. An incident report will need to be completed.

Transferring a client from bed to wheelchair

Equipment: wheelchair, transfer belt, nonskid footwear, folded blanket

1. Wash your hands.

2. Explain the procedure to the client, speaking clearly, slowly, and directly. Maintain face-to-face contact whenever possible.

3. Provide privacy if the client desires it. Check the area to be certain it is uncluttered and safe.

4. Place wheelchair at the head of the bed, facing foot of the bed, or at the foot of bed, facing head of bed. The arm of the wheelchair should be almost touching the bed. It should be placed on client's stronger, or unaffected, side.

5. Remove both wheelchair foot-rests close to the bed.

6. Lock wheelchair wheels.

7. If bed is adjustable, raise the head of the bed. Adjust bed level to lowest position. If bed is movable, lock bed wheels.

8. Assist client to sitting position with feet flat on the floor. Let client sit for a few minutes to adjust to change in position.

9. Put nonskid footwear on client and fasten securely.

10. Stand in front of client. Stand with feet about shoulder-width apart. Bend your knees.

11. Place the transfer belt around client's waist over clothing (not on bare skin). Tighten the buckle until it is snug. Leave enough room to insert flat fingers/hand comfortably under the belt. Check to make sure that skin or skin folds are not caught under the belt. Grasp the belt securely on both sides, with hands in upward position.

12. Provide instructions to allow client to help with transfer, such as the following: "When you start to stand, push with your hands against the bed." "Once standing, if you're able, you can take small steps in the direction of the chair." "Once standing, reach for the chair with your stronger hand."

13. With your legs, brace (support) client's lower legs to prevent slipping. This can be done by placing one or both of your knees in front of the client's knees.

14. Count to three to alert client. On three, with hands still grasping the transfer belt on both sides and moving upward, slowly help client to stand. Make sure the client is not dizzy before proceeding.

15. Tell the client to take small steps in the direction of the chair while turning his back toward it. If more help is needed, help the client pivot (turn) to stand in front of wheelchair with back of client's legs against wheelchair (Fig. 4-8).

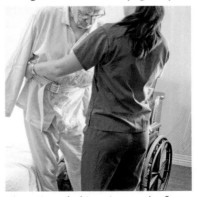

Fig. 4-8. *Help him pivot to the front of the wheelchair.*

16. Ask the client to put hands on wheelchair armrests if able. When the chair is touching the back of the client's legs, help him lower himself into the chair.

17. Reposition client so that his hips touch the back of the wheelchair seat.

18. Attach footrests. Place the client's feet on the footrests.

Check that the client is in proper alignment. Gently remove the transfer belt. Place a folded blanket over the client's lap as appropriate.

19. Wash your hands.

20. Document the procedure and your observations. How did the client feel or appear during the transfer? How much assistance was required?

A slide or transfer board may be used to help transfer clients who are unable to bear weight on their legs. Slide boards can be used for almost any transfer that involves moving from one sitting position to another (for example, from bed to chair). Slide boards should not be used against bare skin.

Helping a client transfer using a slide board

1. Follow steps 1 through 9 of the procedure for transferring a client from a bed to a wheelchair.

2. Have the client lean away from transfer side to take the weight off her thigh (Fig. 4-9). Place one end of the slide board under the buttocks and thigh. Take care not to pinch the client's skin between the bed and the board. Place the other end of the sliding board on the surface to which the client is transferring.

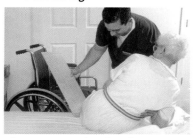

Fig. 4-9. Have the client lean away from the transfer side before placing the slide board.

3. If the client is able, have her push up with her hands and scoot herself across the board. Stay close so you can provide support if needed. Allow the client to do all she can for herself.

4. If the client needs assistance, stand in front of her and brace your knees against her knees to keep them from buckling during the transfer. Make sure your back is straight.

5. Get as close to the client as possible and have her lean into you as you grasp the transfer belt from behind. Lean back with your knees bent. Using your legs rather than your back, pull the client up slightly and toward you to help her scoot across the board (Fig. 4-10).

6. Complete the transfer in two or three lifting and scooting movements. Never drag the client across the board. Friction

from the client's skin dragging across the slide board can cause skin breakdown that can lead to pressure ulcers.

7. After the client is safely transferred, remove the slide board. Make sure the client is positioned safely and comfortably.

8. Wash your hands.

9. Document the procedure and any observations. How did the client feel or appear during the transfer? How much assistance was required?

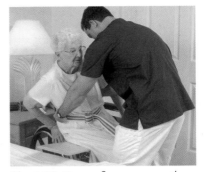

Fig. 4-10. Keep a firm grasp on the transfer belt as you help the client to scoot across the board.

HHAs may assist clients with many types of transfers using mechanical, or hydraulic, lifts. This equipment helps prevent injury to HHAs and clients. There are many different types of mechanical lifts. Using these lifts requires special training. HHAs should not use equipment they have not been trained to use, as this could cause injury. They should always ask for help if there is anything they do not understand about lift equipment.

Transferring a client using a mechanical lift

Equipment: wheelchair or chair, lifting partner (if available), mechanical lift

1. Wash your hands.

2. Explain the procedure to the client, speaking clearly, slowly, and directly. Maintain face-to-face contact whenever possible.

3. Provide privacy if the client desires it.

4. If bed is movable, lock bed wheels.

5. Position wheelchair next to bed. Lock brakes.

6. Check the sling for any fraying or tears. If the sling is damaged, do not use it. Report this to the supervisor.

7. Help the client turn to one side of the bed. Position the sling under the client, with the edge next to the client's back. Fanfold if necessary. Make the bottom of the sling even with the client's knees. Help the client roll back to the middle of the bed, and then spread out the fanfolded edge of the sling.

8. Roll the mechanical lift to bedside. Make sure the base is opened to its widest point. Push the base of the lift under the bed.

9. Place the overhead bar directly over the client.

10. With the client lying on his back, attach one set of straps to each side of the sling. Attach one set of straps to the overhead bar. If available, have a lifting partner support the client at the head, shoulders, and at the knees while being lifted.

The client's arms should be folded across his chest (Fig. 4-11). If the device has **S** hooks, they should face away from the client.

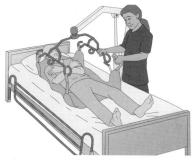

Fig. 4-11. With the client's arms folded across his chest, attach the straps to the sling.

11. Following manufacturer's instructions, raise the client two inches above the bed. Pause a moment for the client to gain balance.

12. Have lifting partner support and guide the client's body while you roll the lift so that the client is positioned over the chair or wheelchair (Fig. 4-12).

13. Slowly lower the client into the chair or wheelchair. Push down gently on the client's knees to help the client into a sitting, rather than reclining, position.

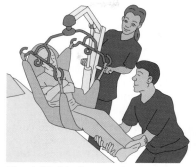

Fig. 4-12. Having another person help to support and guide the client promotes safety during the transfer and lessens the chance of injury.

14. Undo the straps from the overhead bar to the sling. Remove sling or leave in place; follow agency policy.

15. Be sure the client is seated comfortably and correctly in the chair or wheelchair.

16. Wash your hands.

17. Document the procedure and any observations. How did the client tolerate the transfer? Were there any problems? Did the equipment operate properly?

Ambulation is walking. A client who is **ambulatory** is one who can get out of bed and walk. Many older clients are ambulatory, but need help to walk safely. Several tools, including gait belts, canes, walkers, and crutches, assist with ambulation.

Assisting a client to ambulate

Equipment: gait belt, nonskid shoes

1. Wash your hands.

2. Explain the procedure to the client, speaking clearly, slowly, and directly. Maintain face-to-face contact whenever possible.

3. Provide privacy if the client desires it.

4. If the bed is adjustable, adjust bed to lowest position. Lock bed wheels. Assist client to sitting position with feet flat on the floor.

5. Before ambulating, put nonskid footwear on client and securely fasten.

6. Stand in front of and face the client. Place your feet about shoulder-width apart.

7. Place gait belt around client's waist over clothing (not on bare skin). Grasp belt securely on both sides.

8. If client is unable to stand without help, brace (support) the client's lower extremities. This can be done by placing one of your knees against the client's knee. It can also be done by placing both of your knees against both of the client's knees (Fig. 4-13). Bend your knees.

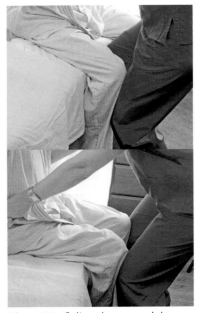

Fig. 4-13. If client has a weak knee, either brace it against your knee, as in top photo, or use both knees to brace the client's knees, as in bottom photo.

9. Hold the client close to your center of gravity. Provide instructions to allow client to help with standing. Tell the client to lean forward, push down on the bed with his hands, and stand on the count of three. On three, with hands still grasping the gait belt on both sides and moving upward, slowly help client to stand. Make sure the client is not dizzy before proceeding.

10. Walk slightly behind and to one side of client for the full ordered distance, while holding onto the gait belt (Fig. 4-14). If the client has a weaker side, stand on the weaker side. Ask client to look forward, not down at the floor, during ambulation.

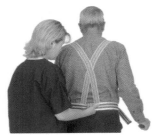

Fig. 4-14. Walk behind and to one side while holding onto the gait belt when assisting with ambulation.

11. After ambulation, help client to the bed or chair. Remove gait belt. Check that client is in proper alignment.

12. Leave bed in lowest position.

13. Wash your hands.

14. Document the procedure and your observations. How far did the client walk? How did the client appear or say he felt while walking? How much help did you give?

Clients who have difficulty walking may use canes, walkers, or crutches to help themselves.

Guidelines: Cane or Walker Use

G   Make sure the walker or cane is in proper condition. It must have rubber tips on the bottom. The tips should not be cracked. Walkers may have wheels. If so, roll the walker to make sure the wheels are moving properly.

G   Be sure the client is wearing securely fastened nonskid shoes.

G   When using a cane, have the client place it on his stronger side.

G   When using a walker, have the client place both hands on the walker. The walker should not be over-extended. It should be placed no more than six inches in front of the client.

G   Stay near the client on the weaker side.

Assisting with ambulation for a client using a cane, walker, or crutches

Equipment: gait belt, nonskid shoes, cane, walker, or crutches

1. Wash your hands.

2. Explain the procedure to the client, speaking clearly, slowly, and directly. Maintain face-to-face contact whenever possible.

3. Provide privacy if the client desires it.

4. If the bed is adjustable, adjust bed to lowest position. Lock bed wheels. Assist client to sitting position with feet flat on the floor.

5. Before ambulating, put nonskid footwear on client and securely fasten.

6. Stand in front of and face the client. Place your feet about shoulder-width apart.

7. Place gait belt around client's waist over clothing (not on bare skin). Grasp belt securely on both sides.

8. If client is unable to stand without help, brace (support) the client's lower extremities (see previous procedure). Bend your knees. Help the client to stand as described in previous procedure.

9. Help as needed with ambulation.

a. *Cane*: Client places cane about six inches, or a comfortable distance, in front of his stronger leg. He brings weaker leg even with cane. He then brings stronger leg forward slightly ahead of cane (Fig. 4-15). Repeat.

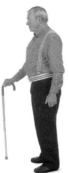

Fig. 4-15. *The cane moves in front of the stronger leg first.*

b. *Walker*: Client picks up or rolls the walker. He places it about six inches, or a comfortable distance, in front of him. All four feet or wheels of the walker should be on the ground before client steps forward to the walker. The walker should not be moved again until the client has moved both feet forward and is steady (Fig. 4-16). The client should never put his feet ahead of the walker.

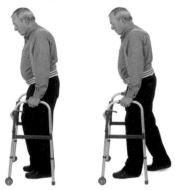

Fig. 4-16. *The walker can be moved after the client is steady and both feet are forward.*

c. *Crutches*: Client should be fitted for crutches and taught to use them correctly by a physical therapist or a nurse. The client may use the crutches several different ways. No matter how they are used, the client's weight should be on his hands and arms. Weight should not be on the underarm area (Fig. 4-17).

10. Walk slightly behind and to one side of client. Stay on the weak side if the client has one. Hold the gait belt.

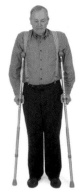

Fig. 4-17. *When using crutches, weight should be on the hands and arms, not on the underarms.*

11. Watch for obstacles in the client's path. Ask the client to look forward, not down at the floor, during ambulation.

12. Encourage the client to rest if tired. When a person is tired, it increases the chance of a fall. Let the client set the pace. Discuss how far he plans to go based on the care plan.

13. After ambulation, help client to the bed or chair. Remove gait belt. Check that client is in proper alignment.

14. Leave bed in lowest position.

15. Wash your hands.

16. Document the procedure and your observations. How did the client feel or appear while walking? How far did the client walk? How much help did the client need?

Range of Motion Exercises

Exercise helps people regain strength and mobility. It prevents disabilities from developing. People who are in bed for long periods of time are more likely to develop muscle atrophy or contractures. When atrophy occurs, the muscle wastes away, decreases in size, and becomes weak. When a contracture develops, the muscle or tendon shortens, becomes inflexible, and "freezes" in position. Contractures and atrophy are generally caused by immobility and result in a loss of ability. **Range of motion (ROM)** exercises put a joint through its full arc of motion. The goal of these exercises is to decrease or prevent contractures or atrophy, improve strength, and increase circulation.

Active range of motion (AROM) exercises are performed by a client himself, without help. The HHA's role in AROM exercises is to encourage the client. Active assisted range of motion (AAROM) exercises are performed by the client with some help and support from the HHA. Passive range of motion (PROM) exercises are used when clients are not able to move on their own. An HHA performs these exercises without the client's help. Range of motion exercises are specific for each body area. They include these movements (Fig. 4-18):

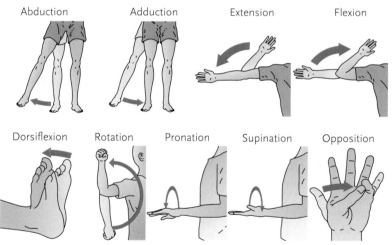

Fig. 4-18. The different range of motion body movements.

- **Abduction**: moving a body part away from the midline of the body
- **Adduction**: moving a body part toward the midline of the body
- **Extension**: straightening a body part
- **Flexion**: bending a body part
- **Dorsiflexion**: bending backward
- **Rotation**: turning a joint
- **Pronation**: turning downward

- **Supination**: turning upward
- **Opposition**: touching the thumb to any other finger

HHAs will not perform ROM exercises without an order from a doctor, nurse, or physical therapist. The HHA will repeat each exercise three to five times, once or twice a day, working on both sides of the body. When doing ROM exercises, the HHA should begin at the client's shoulders and work down the body. The upper extremities (arms) should be exercised before the lower extremities (legs). The HHA should give support above and below the joint. The joints should be moved gently, slowly, and smoothly. The HHA should stop the exercises if the client complains of pain and report the pain to the supervisor.

Assisting with passive range of motion exercises

1. Wash your hands.

2. Explain the procedure to the client, speaking clearly, slowly, and directly. Maintain face-to-face contact whenever possible.

3. Provide privacy if the client desires it.

4. If the bed is adjustable, adjust bed to a safe level, usually waist high. If the bed is movable, lock bed wheels.

5. Position the client lying supine—flat on her back—on the bed. Use proper alignment.

6. While supporting the limbs, move all joints gently, slowly, and smoothly through the range of motion to the point of resistance. Repeat each exercise at least three times. Stop if any pain occurs.

7. *Shoulder:* Support the client's arm at the elbow and wrist while performing ROM for the shoulder. Place one hand under the elbow and the other hand under the wrist. Raise the straightened arm from the side position upward toward head to ear level. Return arm down to side of the body (extension/flexion) (Fig. 4-19).

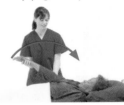

Fig. 4-19. Raise the straightened arm upward toward head to ear level and return it to the side of the body.

Move straightened arm away from side of body to shoulder level. Return arm to side of body (abduction/adduction) (Fig. 4-20).

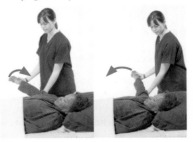

Fig. 4-20. Move straightened arm away from side of body to shoulder level and return arm to side.

8. *Elbow*: Hold the client's wrist with one hand and the elbow with the other hand. Bend the elbow so that the hand touches the shoulder on that same side (flexion). Straighten arm (extension) (Fig. 4-21).

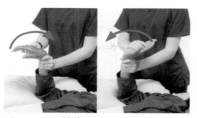

Fig. 4-23. *While supporting the wrist, gently bend the hand down and then backward.*

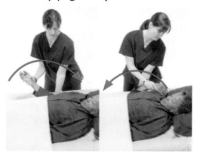

Fig. 4-21. *Bend the elbow so that the hand touches the shoulder on the same side. Then straighten the arm.*

Exercise the forearm by moving it so palm is facing downward (pronation) and then the palm is facing upward (supination) (Fig. 4-22).

Turn the hand in the direction of the thumb (radial flexion). Then turn the hand in the direction of the little finger (ulnar flexion) (Fig. 4-24).

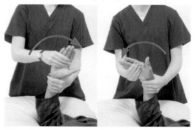

Fig. 4-24. *Turn the hand in the direction of the thumb, then turn it in the direction of the little finger.*

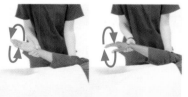

Fig. 4-22. *Exercise the forearm so that the palm is facing downward and then upward.*

10. *Thumb*: Move the thumb away from the index finger (abduction). Move the thumb back next to the index finger (adduction) (Fig. 4-25).

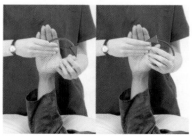

9. *Wrist*: Hold the wrist with one hand. Use the fingers of the other hand to help move the joint through the motions. Bend the hand down (flexion); bend the hand backward (dorsiflexion) (Fig. 4-23).

Fig. 4-25. *Move the thumb away from the index finger and then back to the index finger.*

Touch each fingertip with the thumb (opposition) (Fig. 4-26).

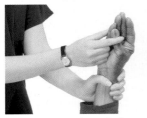

Fig. 4-26. Touch each fingertip with the thumb.

Bend thumb into the palm (flexion) and out to the side (extension) (Fig. 4-27).

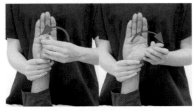

Fig. 4-27. Bend the thumb into the palm and then out to the side.

11. *Fingers*: Make the hand into a fist (flexion). Gently straighten out the fist (extension) (Fig. 4-28).

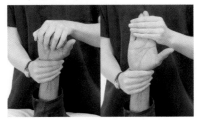

Fig. 4-28. Make the fingers into a fist and then gently straighten out the fist.

Spread the fingers and the thumb far apart from each other (abduction). Bring the fingers back next to each other (adduction) (Fig. 4-29).

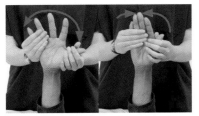

Fig. 4-29. Spread the fingers and thumb far apart from each other and then bring them back next to each other.

12. *Hip*. Support the leg by placing one hand under the knee and one under the ankle. Straighten the leg and raise it gently upward. Move the leg away from the other leg (abduction). Move the leg toward the other leg (adduction) (Fig. 4-30).

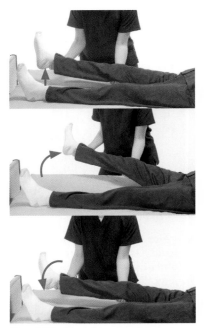

Fig. 4-30. Straighten the leg and gently raise it. Move the leg away from the other leg and then back toward the other leg.

Gently turn the leg inward (internal rotation). Turn the leg outward (external rotation) (Fig. 4-31).

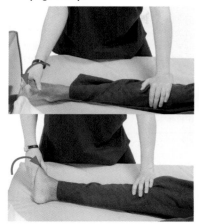

Fig. 4-31. Gently turn the leg inward and then outward.

13. *Knees*: Support the leg under the knee and ankle while performing ROM for the knee. Bend the leg to the point of resistance (flexion). Return leg to client's normal position (extension) (Fig. 4-32).

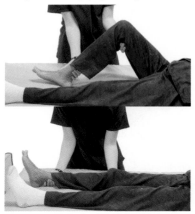

Fig. 4-32. Gently bend the knee to the point of resistance and return the leg to its normal position.

14. *Ankle*: Support the foot and ankle close to the bed while performing ROM for the ankle. Push/pull foot up toward the head (dorsiflexion). Push/pull foot down, with the toes pointed down (plantar flexion) (Fig. 4-33).

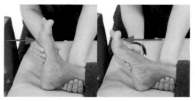

Fig. 4-33. Push the foot up toward the head and then push it back down.

Turn inside of the foot inward toward the body (supination). Bend the sole of the foot so that it faces away from the body (pronation) (Fig. 4-34).

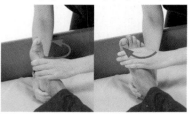

Fig. 4-34. Turn inside of foot inward, toward the body, and then bend it to face away from the body.

15. *Toes*: Curl and straighten the toes (flexion and extension) (Fig. 4-35).

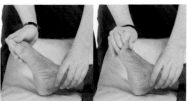

Fig. 4-35. Curl and straighten the toes.

Gently spread the toes apart (abduction) (Fig. 4-36).

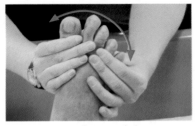

Fig. 4-36. *Gently spread the toes apart.*

16. Return client to comfortable position.

17. Wash your hands.

18. Document the procedure. Note any decrease in range of motion or any pain experienced by the client. Notify the supervisor or the physical therapist if you find increased stiffness or physical resistance. Resistance may be a sign that a contracture is developing.

Skin Care

Clients who have restricted mobility have greater risk of skin deterioration at pressure points. Pressure points are areas of the body that bear much of its weight. Pressure points are mainly located at bony prominences. Bony prominences are areas of the body where the bone lies close to the skin. The skin here is at a much higher risk for skin breakdown. These areas include elbows, shoulder blades, tailbone, hip and knees (inner and outer parts), ankles, heels, toes, and the backs of the neck and head. Other areas at risk are the ears, the area under the breasts or scrotum, the area between the folds of the buttocks or abdomen, and skin between the legs (Fig. 4-37).

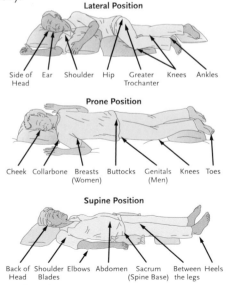

Fig. 4-37. *Pressure ulcer danger zones.*

The pressure on these areas reduces circulation, decreasing the amount of oxygen the cells receive. Warmth and moisture also add to skin breakdown. Once the surface of the skin is weakened, pathogens can invade and cause infection. When infection occurs, the healing process slows.

When the skin begins to break down, it becomes pale, white, or a reddened color. Darker skin may look purple. The client may also feel tingling or burning in the area. This discoloration does not go away, even when the client's position is changed. If pressure is allowed to continue, the area will further break down. The resulting wound is called a **pressure ulcer**, pressure sore, bed sore, or decubitus ulcer. If caught early, a break in the skin can heal fairly quickly without other problems. Once a pressure ulcer forms, it can get bigger and deeper and become infected. Pressure ulcers are painful and are difficult to heal. They can lead to life-threatening infections. Prevention is very important.

Observing and Reporting: Client's Skin

- Pale, white, reddened, or purple areas
- Blisters or bruises
- Complaints of tingling, warmth, or burning of the skin
- Dry or flaking skin
- Itching or scratching
- Rash or any skin discoloration
- Swelling
- Fluid or blood draining from skin
- Broken skin
- Wounds or ulcers on the skin
- Changes in wound or ulcer (size, depth, drainage, color, odor)
- Redness or broken skin between toes or around toenails

In darker complexions, also look for

- Any change in the feel of the tissue; any change in the appearance of the skin, such as the "orange-peel" look; a purplish hue; or extremely dry, crust-like areas that might be covering a tissue break

Guidelines: Basic Skin Care

G   Report any changes you observe in a client's skin.

G   Provide regular, daily care for skin to keep it clean and dry. Check the skin daily, even when complete baths are not given or taken every day. Always check the client's skin when bathing.

G   Reposition immobile clients often (at least every two hours).

G   Give frequent and thorough skin care as often as needed for incontinent clients. Change clothing and linens often as well.

G   Do not scratch or irritate the skin in any way. Keep rough, scratchy fabrics away from the client's skin. Report to your supervisor if a client wears shoes that cause blisters or sores.

G   Massage the skin often. Use light, circular strokes to increase circulation. Use little or no pressure on bony areas. Do not massage a white, red, or purple area or put any pressure on it. Massage the healthy skin and tissue around the area.

G   Be gentle during transfers. Avoid pulling or tearing fragile skin.

G   Clients who are overweight may have poor circulation and extra folds of skin. Pay careful attention to the skin under the folds. Keep it clean and dry. Report signs of skin irritation.

G   Encourage well-balanced meals and plenty of fluids. Proper nutrition is important for keeping skin healthy.

G   Keep plastic or rubber materials from coming into contact with the client's skin. These materials prevent air from circulating, which causes the skin to sweat.

G   Follow the care plan. It may include instructions about special skin care, such as washing the skin with a special soap.

For clients who are not mobile or cannot change positions easily:

G   Keep the bottom sheet tight and free from wrinkles. Keep the bed free from crumbs. Keep clothing or gowns free of wrinkles, too.

G   Do not pull the client across sheets during transfers or repositioning. This can cause **shearing**, which can lead to skin breakdown.

G   Place a sheepskin or bed pad under the back and buttocks to absorb moisture. It can also protect the skin from irritating bed linens. Sheepskin covers are also available for wheelchairs.

G   Relieve pressure under bony prominences. Use a pillow under the calves so that heels are elevated ("floating").

G   A bed or chair can be made softer with flotation pads.

G   Use a bed cradle to keep top sheets from rubbing the client's skin.

G   Reposition clients seated in chairs or wheelchairs at least every hour if they cannot change positions easily.

Comfort Measures

Many positioning devices are available to help make clients safer and more comfortable. Some can be inexpensively made in the client's home.

Guidelines: Positioning Devices

G   Backrests provide support. They can be regular pillows, cardboard or wood covered by pillows, or special wedge-shaped foam pillows.

G   Bed cradles or foot cradles are used to keep the bed covers from resting on a client's legs and feet. Metal frames that work like a tent when the bed covers are over them can be purchased. A cardboard box can be used as a bed cradle by placing the client's feet inside the box underneath the covers. The box should be at least two inches above the toes.

G   Bed tables are available commercially. You can also make one by cutting openings in each of the longer sides of a sturdy cardboard box.

G   Draw sheets may be placed under clients who cannot help with turning, lifting, or moving up in bed. Draw sheets help prevent skin damage from shearing. A regular bed sheet folded in half can be used as a draw sheet.

G   Footboards are padded boards placed against the client's feet to keep them properly aligned and to help prevent **foot drop**. Footboards are also used to keep bed covers off the feet. Rolled blankets or pillows can also be used as foot boards.

G   Handrolls are cloth-covered or rubber items that keep the fingers from curling tightly. A rolled washcloth, gauze bandage, or a rubber ball placed inside the palm may be used to keep the hand in a natural position. Handrolls can help prevent finger, hand, or wrist contractures.

G   An **orthotic device**, or orthosis, is a device that helps support and align a limb and improve its functioning. It may be prescribed to help keep a client's joints in the correct position. Orthoses also help prevent or correct deformities. Splints are a type of orthotic device. Splints and the skin area around them should be cleaned at least once daily and as needed. Follow the care plan.

G   Trochanter rolls are rolled towels or blankets used to keep the client's hips from turning outward.

G   Pillows between the legs from knees to ankles, while in the lateral position, can help keep the spine, hips, and knees in the proper position. They ease pain in the back, leg, hip, and knee areas.

A back rub can help clients relax and make them more comfortable. It can also increase circulation. Back rubs are often given after baths.

Giving a back rub

Equipment: cotton blanket or towel, lotion

1. Wash your hands.

2. Explain the procedure to the client, speaking clearly, slowly, and directly. Maintain face-to-face contact whenever possible.

3. Provide privacy for the client.

4. If the bed is adjustable, adjust bed to a safe working level, usually waist high. Lower the head of the bed. If the bed is movable, lock bed wheels.

5. Position client lying on his side or stomach. Cover client with a cotton blanket or towel. Fold back bed covers. Expose the back to the top of the buttocks. Back rubs can also be given with the client sitting up.

6. Warm the lotion by putting bottle in warm water for five minutes. Run your hands under warm water. Pour lotion on your hands. Rub them together. Always put the lotion on your hands first, rather than directly on the client's skin.

7. Place your hands on each side of the upper part of the buttocks. Use the full palm of each hand. Make long, smooth upward strokes with both hands. Move along each side of the spine, up to the shoulders (Fig. 4-38). Circle your hands outward. Move back along the outer edges of the back. At buttocks, make another circle and move your hands back up to the shoulders. Without taking your hands off the client's skin, repeat this motion for three to five minutes.

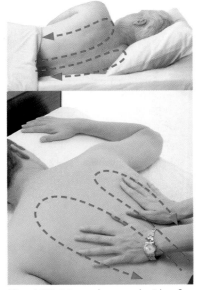

Fig. 4-38. *Move along each side of the spine, up to the shoulders. Upward strokes help release muscle tension.*

8. Knead with the first two fingers and thumb of each hand. Place them at the base of the spine. Move upward together along each side of the spine, applying gentle downward pressure with the fingers and thumbs. Follow the same direction as with the long smooth strokes, circling at shoulders and buttocks.

9. Gently massage bony areas (spine, shoulder blades, hip bones) with circular motions of your fingertips. If any of these areas is pale, white, or red, massage around it rather than on it. Discoloration indicates that the skin is already irritated and fragile.

10. Let the client know when you are almost through. Finish with some long smooth strokes.

11. Dry the back if extra lotion remains on it.

12. Remove the cotton blanket and towel.

13. Help the client get dressed. Help the client into a comfortable position. If you raised an adjustable bed, return it to its lowest position.

14. Store supplies, and place soiled clothing and linens in the hamper.

15. Wash your hands.

16. Document the procedure and your observations. Did the client appear comfortable during the back rub? Did you observe any discolored areas or broken skin?

Personal Care Procedures

People working as CNAs or HHAs have learned personal care skills already. This section will serve as a review of the basic procedures most often provided for clients in their homes. Clients should be encouraged to do as much of the care by themselves as possible. This promotes independence.

Hygiene is the term used to describe ways to keep bodies clean and healthy. Bathing and brushing teeth are two examples. Grooming refers to practices like caring for fingernails and hair. Hygiene and grooming activities, as well as dressing, eating, transferring, and toileting are called **activities of daily living (ADLs)**. Personal care includes such activities as bathing, perineal care (care of the genital and anal area), toileting, mouth care, shampooing and combing the hair, nail care, shaving, dressing, eating, walking, transferring, and changing bed linens.

Before beginning a task, the HHA should explain to the client exactly what she will be doing. Explaining care to a client is not only his legal right, but it may also help lessen anxiety. The HHA should ask if he would like to use the bathroom or bedpan first. She should provide privacy for the client. The client should be allowed to make as many decisions as possible about when, where, and how a procedure is done. This promotes dignity and independence. If the client appears tired during a procedure, the HHA should stop so the client can take a short rest. After care, the HHA should always ask if the client would like anything else.

Observing and Reporting: Personal Care

O/R   Skin color, temperature, redness

O/R   Mobility

°/ℝ Flexibility

°/ℝ Comfort level, or complaints of pain or discomfort

°/ℝ Strength and the ability to perform self-care and ADLs

°/ℝ Mental and emotional state

°/ℝ Client complaints

Bathing

Bathing promotes health and well-being. It removes perspiration, dirt, oil, and dead skin cells from the skin. Bathing can also be relaxing. The bed bath is an excellent time for moving arms and legs and increasing circulation. Many agencies have rules against HHAs helping clients into the bathtub. These rules are for the client's safety as well as the home health aide's. HHAs should follow their agency's policies and procedures. Some clients may be embarrassed or uncomfortable with someone helping them bathe. The HHA should be sensitive to this and provide privacy. She should be professional and respectful.

Guidelines: Bathing

G The face, hands, axillae (underarms), and perineum should be washed every day. A complete bath or shower can be taken every other day or less often. Older skin produces less perspiration and oil. Elderly people with dry, fragile skin should bathe only once or twice a week. This helps prevent further dryness and itchy skin. Be gentle with the skin when bathing clients.

G Before any bathing task, make sure the room is warm enough.

G Remove any loose rugs that do not have slip-resistant, rubber backings.

G Be familiar with available safety and assistive devices.

G Never leave an elderly person or young child alone in the bathtub. Gather supplies before giving a bath so the client is not left alone.

G Before bathing, make sure the water temperature is safe and comfortable. Test the water temperature with a thermometer or against the inside of your wrist to make sure it is not too hot. Then have the client test the water temperature. The client is best able to choose a comfortable water temperature.

G Make sure all soap is removed from the skin before completing the bath.

G Do not use bath oils, lotions, or powders in showers or tubs. They make surfaces slippery.

Helping a client transfer to the bathtub

You may have to adapt this procedure to work with your clients' different strength levels.

Equipment: chair, transfer belt (if appropriate), shirt or robe to wear under transfer belt, slide board (if appropriate), tub or shower chair, bath supplies (as listed in next procedure)

1. Wash your hands.

2. Explain the procedure to the client, speaking clearly, slowly, and directly. Maintain face-to-face contact whenever possible.

3. Help the client to the bathroom.

4. Provide privacy for the client.

5. Seat the client in a chair facing the bathtub and centered between the grab bars. If using a wheelchair, lock brakes and raise footrests (Fig. 4-39).

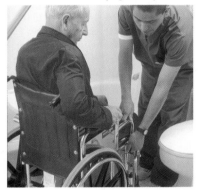

Fig. 4-39. *Lock the wheelchair before beginning to transfer a client.*

6. Ask the client to place one leg at a time over the sides of the tub.

7. Have client hold on to the grab bars or the edge of the tub to bring himself to a sitting position on the edge of the tub (Fig. 4-40). A slide board may also be used to help the client move from the chair to the tub.

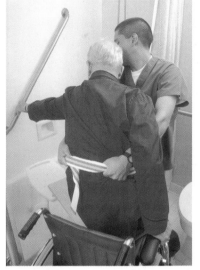

Fig. 4-40. *Have client hold onto grab bars while moving him into the tub. Keep your back straight and your knees slightly bent while assisting with the move.*

8. Help the client lower himself into the tub or onto the tub chair (bath bench) while holding on to the edge of the tub or grab bars. If necessary, assist by holding him around the waist or by having him wear a transfer belt. If using a transfer belt to get in and out of the tub, the client will need to wear a shirt or robe while transferring, so the belt is not placed directly against his skin. When he is in the tub, place supplies within easy reach (Fig. 4-41).

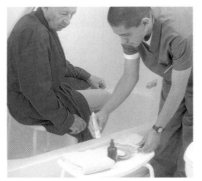

Fig. 4-41. *Keep bathing supplies close to client during shower or tub bath.*

9. Reverse this procedure to help the client out of the tub when the bath is over. If the client has trouble getting out of the tub, help him to his hands and knees. From that position, he can use the grab bar or the edge of the tub to help pull himself up. You can also help by putting the transfer belt back on the client (over a robe).

10. Wash your hands.

11. Document the procedure and your observations.

Clients who can get out of bed to take a shower or bath will need different assistance and supervision. The care plan will include necessary instructions.

Helping the ambulatory client take a shower or tub bath

Equipment: two bath towels, washcloth, soap or other cleanser, bath thermometer (if available), rubber bath mat, tub or shower chair (if appropriate), table for bath supplies and bell (for clients who bathe without assistance), non-skid bath rug, deodorant, lotion and other toiletries, clean clothes or a robe, shoes or nonskid slippers, gloves

1. Wash your hands.

2. Explain the procedure to the client, speaking clearly, slowly, and directly. Maintain face-to-face contact whenever possible.

3. Clean tub or shower if necessary. Place rubber mat on tub or shower floor. Set up tub or shower chair. Place nonskid bath rug on the floor next to the tub or shower.

4. Provide privacy for the client.

5. Fill the tub halfway with warm water or adjust the shower water temperature. Turn on cold water first, then add hot water. This helps reduce the risk of burns. Test water temperature with the bath thermometer or the inside of your wrist to see if it is comfortable. Water temperature should be no higher than 105°F. Have the client test water temperature to see if it is comfortable. Adjust if necessary.

6. Put on gloves.

7. Ask the client to undress, and assist as needed. Help client transfer to bathtub or step in the shower.

8. If the care plan allows you to leave the client to bathe alone, place the bathing supplies on a small table within the client's reach. Place a bell or other signal on the table (Fig. 4-42). Tell the client to signal when you are needed. Ask the client not

to add more hot or warm water and not to remain in the tub more than 20 minutes. Do not lock the bathroom door. Check on your client every five minutes. If the client is weak or confused, remain in the bathroom. Otherwise, you can make the client's bed while he is in the tub.

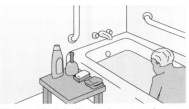

Fig. 4-42. A bell or other signal provides a way for the client to communicate that he needs you.

9. For a shower, stay with the client and assist with washing hard-to-reach areas. Observe for signs of fatigue.

10. If the client needs more assistance in the bath or shower, help him wash himself. Always wash from clean areas to dirty areas so you do not spread dirt into areas that have already been washed. Make sure all soap is rinsed off so the client's skin does not become dry or irritated.

11. Assist the client with shampooing hair, if necessary (see procedure later in chapter). Make sure all shampoo is rinsed out of hair.

12. When the bath or shower is finished, help the client get out of the tub. Wrap him in a towel. Have the client sit in a chair or

on the toilet seat, and provide him with another towel for drying himself (Fig. 4-43). Offer assistance in drying hard-to-reach places. The client may need help applying powder, deodorant, or lotion. If necessary, help the client get dressed.

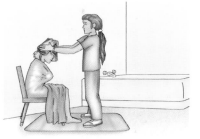

Fig. 4-43. Give the client any needed assistance when drying herself.

13. If your client is tired after the bath or shower, help him back to the bed. Other personal care, such as mouth care, can be done later or while the client is in bed.

14. Clean the tub and place soiled laundry (towels, washcloths, dirty clothes) in the hamper.

15. Remove and discard gloves.

16. Wash your hands.

17. Store supplies.

18. Document the procedure and your observations. Did you observe any redness or whiteness on the skin? Was there any broken skin? How did the client tolerate bathing or showering? Has there been a change in the client's abilities since the last bath or shower?

Giving a complete bed bath

Equipment: soft cotton blanket or large towel, bath basin, soap, bath thermometer (if available), 2-4 washcloths, 2-4 bath towels, clean clothes, 2 pairs of gloves, lotion, deodorant, brush or comb, orangewood stick or nail brush (if available)

When bathing, move client's body gently and naturally. Avoid force and over-extension of limbs and joints.

1. Wash your hands.

2. Explain the procedure to the client, speaking clearly, slowly, and directly. Maintain face-to-face contact whenever possible.

3. Provide privacy for the client. Be sure the room is a comfortable temperature and there are no drafts.

4. If the bed is adjustable, adjust bed to a safe level, usually waist high. If the bed is movable, lock bed wheels.

5. Ask client to remove eyeglasses and jewelry and put them in a safe place. Offer a bedpan or urinal for the client to use before the bath.

6. Place a soft cotton blanket or towel over client (Fig. 4-44). Ask him to hold on to it as you remove or fold back top bedding. Remove gown, while keeping client covered with blanket. Place gown in hamper.

7. Fill the basin with warm water. Test water temperature with a bath thermometer or against the inside of your wrist. Water temperature should be no higher than 105°F. Have the client test water temperature to see if it is comfortable. Adjust if necessary. The water will cool quickly. Change the water when it becomes too cool, soapy, or dirty.

8. Put on gloves.

9. Ask the client to participate in washing. Help him do this when needed.

10. Uncover only one part of the body at a time. Place a towel under the part being washed.

11. Wash, rinse, and dry one part of the body at a time. Start at the head. Work down, and complete the front first. When washing, use a clean area of the washcloth for each stroke.

    Eyes, Face, Ears, and Neck: Wash face with wet washcloth (no soap). Begin with the eye farther away from you. Wash inner to outer area (Fig. 4-45). Use a different area of the washcloth for each stroke. Wash the face from the middle outward. Use firm but gentle strokes. Wash the ears and behind the ears. Wash the neck. Rinse and pat dry.

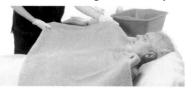

Fig. 4-44. *Cover the client with a cotton blanket before removing top bedding.*

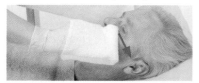

Fig. 4-45. *Wash the eye from the inner to outer area, using a different area of the washcloth for each stroke.*

Arms and Axillae: Remove one arm from under the towel. With a soapy washcloth, wash the upper arm and underarm. Use long strokes from the shoulder down to the wrist. Rinse and pat dry. Repeat for the other arm (Fig. 4-46).

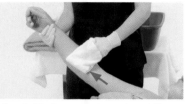

Fig. 4-46. Support the wrist while washing the shoulder, arm, underarm, and elbow.

Hands: Wash one hand in a basin. Clean under the nails with an orangewood stick or nail brush (Fig. 4-47). Rinse and pat dry. Give nail care (see procedure later in this chapter). Repeat for the other hand. Put lotion on the client's elbows and hands if ordered.

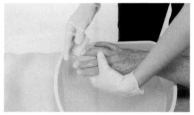

Fig. 4-47. Wash each hand in a basin. Thoroughly clean under the nails with a nail brush.

Chest: Place the towel across the client's chest. Pull the blanket down to the waist. Lift the towel only enough to wash the chest. Rinse it and pat dry. For a female client, wash, rinse, and dry breasts and under breasts. Check the skin in this area for signs of irritation.

Abdomen: Keep towel across chest. Fold the blanket down so that it still covers the pubic area. Wash the abdomen, rinse, and pat dry. If the client has an ostomy, give skin care around the opening (see *Special Procedures* later in this section). Cover with the towel. Pull the cotton blanket up to the client's chin. Remove the towel.

Legs and Feet: Expose one leg. Place a towel under it. Wash the thigh. Use long downward strokes. Rinse and pat dry. Do the same from the knee to the ankle (Fig. 4-48).

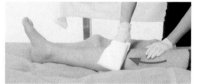

Fig. 4-48. Use long downward strokes when washing the legs.

Place another towel under the foot. Move the basin to the towel. Place the foot into the basin. Wash the foot and between the toes (Fig. 4-49). Rinse foot and pat dry. Make sure areas between toes are dry. Apply lotion to the foot if ordered, especially at the heels. Do not apply lotion between the toes. Repeat steps for the other leg and foot.

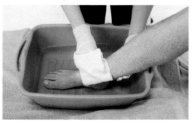

Fig. 4-49. Wash the feet includes cleaning between the toes.

Back: Help client move to the center of the bed. Ask client to turn onto his side so his back is facing you. If the bed has rails, raise the rail on the far side for safety. Fold the blanket away from the back. Place a towel lengthwise next to the back. Wash the neck and back with long, downward strokes (Fig. 4-50). Rinse and pat dry. Apply lotion if ordered.

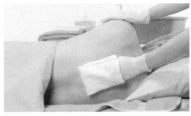

Fig. 4-50. *Wash the back with long, downward strokes.*

12. Place the towel under the buttocks and upper thighs. Help the client turn onto his back. If the client is able to wash his perineal area, place a basin of clean, warm water, a washcloth, and towel within reach. Hand items to the client as needed. If the client wants you to leave the room, remove and discard gloves. Wash your hands. Leave supplies within reach. If the client has a urinary catheter in place, remind him not to pull it.

13. If the client cannot provide perineal care, you will do it. Remove and discard your gloves. Wash your hands and put on clean gloves. Provide privacy at all times.

    Perineal area and buttocks: Change the bath water. Place a towel under the perineal area. Wash, rinse, and dry perineal area. Work from front to back (clean to dirty).

For a female client: Using water and a small amount of soap, wash the perineum from front to back. Use single strokes (Fig. 4-51). Do not wash from the back to the front. This may cause infection. Use a clean area of washcloth or clean washcloth for each stroke.

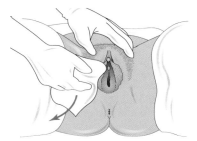

Fig. 4-51. *Always work from front to back when performing perineal care. This helps prevent infection.*

First spread the labia majora, the outside folds of perineal skin that protect the urinary meatus and the vaginal opening. Wipe from front to back on one side with a clean washcloth. Then wipe the other side from front to back, using a clean part of the washcloth. Clean the perineum (area between vagina and anus) last with a front to back motion. Rinse the area thoroughly in the same way. Make sure all soap is removed.

Dry entire perineal area. Move from front to back, using a blotting motion with towel. Ask client to turn on her side. Wash, rinse, and dry buttocks and anal area. Clean the anal area without contaminating the perineal area.

For a male client: If the client is uncircumcised, pull back the foreskin first. Gently push skin towards the base of penis. Hold the penis by the shaft. Wash in a circular motion from the tip down to the base (Fig. 4-52). Use a clean area of washcloth or clean washcloth for each stroke.

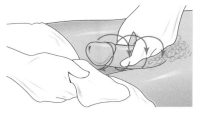

Fig. 4-52. Wash the penis in a circular motion from the tip down to the base.

Thoroughly rinse the penis and pat dry. If client is uncircumcised, gently return foreskin to normal position. Then wash the scrotum and groin. The groin is the area from the pubis (area around the penis and scrotum) to the upper thighs. Rinse and pat dry. Ask the client to turn on his side. Wash, rinse, and dry buttocks and anal area. Clean the anal area without contaminating the perineal area.

14. Cover the client with the cotton blanket.

15. Place soiled washcloths and towels in the hamper or laundry basket. Dispose of the dirty bath water in the toilet. Flush the toilet. Rinse, dry, and store basin.

16. Remove and discard gloves. Wash your hands.

17. If time permits, a bed bath is a good time to give the client a back rub if he wants one.

18. Provide deodorant. Place a towel over the pillow and brush or comb the client's hair (see procedure later in this chapter). Help the client put on clean clothing and get into a comfortable position with proper body alignment. If you raised an adjustable bed, return it to its lowest position.

19. If the client uses a signaling device, place it within reach. Store the bath supplies. If needed, change bed sheets and blanket. Place used bed linens in the hamper or laundry basket.

20. Wash your hands.

21. Document the procedure and your observations. Did you observe any redness, whiteness, or purple areas on the skin? Was there any broken skin? How did the client tolerate bathing? Did the client tell you about any symptoms? Has there been a change in the client's abilities since the last bath?

Grooming

When assisting with grooming, HHAs should always let clients do all they can for themselves. Clients should make as many choices as possible. Clients may have particular ways of grooming themselves. They may have routines. These routines remain important even when people are elderly, sick, or disabled. Some clients may be embarrassed or depressed because they need help with grooming tasks they have performed for themselves all their lives. HHAs can help by being sensitive to this. They should be professional, respectful, and cheerful while assisting clients with grooming.

Clients who can get out of bed may have their hair shampooed in the sink, tub, or shower. For clients who cannot get out of bed, special troughs exist for shampooing hair in bed. Troughs fit under the client's head and neck and have a spout or hose that drains the water into a basin at the side of the bed. A plastic garbage bag formed around a rolled towel can also be used. In addition, there are special types of shampoo that do not require the use of water. Gloves should be worn if a client has open sores on his scalp.

Shampooing hair

Equipment: shampoo, hair conditioner (if requested), 2 bath towels, washcloth, bath thermometer, pitcher or hand-held shower or sink attachment, plastic cup, waterproof pad (for washing hair in bed), cotton blanket (for washing hair in bed), trough and catch basin (for washing hair in bed), chair (for washing hair in sink), large garbage bag or plastic sheet (for washing hair in sink), comb and brush, hair dryer

1. **Wash your hands.**

2. **Explain the procedure to the client, speaking clearly, slowly, and directly. Maintain face-to-face contact whenever possible.**

3. **Provide privacy for the client. Be sure the room is a comfortable temperature and there are no drafts.**

4. **Test water temperature with a bath thermometer or against the inside of your wrist. Water temperature should be no higher than 105°F. Have client check water temperature. Adjust if necessary.**

5. **Position the client and wet the client's hair.**

a. *For washing hair in the sink,* **seat the client in a chair covered with plastic. Use a pillow under the plastic to support the head and neck. Have the client lean her head back toward the sink. Give the client a folded washcloth to hold over her forehead or eyes. Wet hair using a plastic cup, pitcher, or a hand-held sink attachment (Fig. 4-53).**

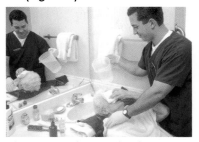

Fig. 4-53. Make sure the client's head and neck are supported and her eyes covered when washing hair in the sink.

b. *For washing hair in the tub,* **have the client tilt her head back. Give the client a folded washcloth to hold over her forehead or eyes. Wet hair using a plastic cup, pitcher, or hand-held shower attachment.**

c. *For washing hair in the shower,* **have the client turn so her back** is toward the showerhead. Ask the client to tilt her head backward. Direct the flow of water over the hair to wet it.

d. *For washing hair in bed,* arrange the supplies within reach on a nearby table. Remove all pillows and place the client in a flat position. If the bed is adjustable, adjust bed to a safe working level, usually waist high. If the bed is movable, lock bed wheels. Place a waterproof pad beneath the client's head and shoulders. Cover the client with the cotton blanket, and fold back the top sheet and regular blankets. Place the trough under the client's head and connect trough to the catch basin. Place one towel across the client's shoulders. Protect the client's eyes with a dry washcloth. Using the pitcher, pour enough water on the client's hair to make it thoroughly wet.

6. Apply a small amount of shampoo to your hands and rub them together. Using both hands, massage the shampoo to a lather in the client's hair. With your fingertips (not fingernails), massage the scalp in a circular motion, from front to back (Fig. 4-54). Do not scratch the scalp.

7. Rinse the hair in the same way you wet it. Rinse until water runs clear. Repeat the shampoo, rinse again, and use conditioner if the client wants it. Be sure to rinse the hair thoroughly to prevent the client's scalp from getting dry and itchy.

8. Wrap the client's hair in a clean towel. If shampooing at the

sink, return the client to an upright position. If shampooing in the bath or shower, assist the client from the tub or shower. If shampooing in bed, remove the trough. Using the washcloth or a face towel, wipe water from the face, head, and neck.

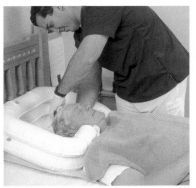

Fig. 4-54. Use your fingertips to work shampoo into a lather. Be gentle so that you do not scratch the scalp.

9. Remove the hair towel and gently rub scalp and hair with the towel. Comb or brush hair (see next procedure).

10. Dry hair with a hair dryer on the low setting. Style hair as the client prefers.

11. Wash and store equipment. Put soiled towels and washcloth in the hamper or laundry basket. If you raised an adjustable bed, return it to its lowest position.

12. Wash your hands.

13. Document the procedure and your observations. How did the client tolerate having her hair washed? Was the client able to help? Have the client's abilities changed since the last time her hair was washed?

HHAs should handle clients' hair very carefully. Because hair thins as people age, pieces of hair can be pulled out of the head while combing or brushing it. HHAs should be gentle when combing or brushing hair.

Combing or brushing hair

Equipment: comb, brush, towel, mirror, hair care items requested by client

Use hair care products that the client prefers for his or her type of hair.

1. Wash your hands.

2. Explain the procedure to the client, speaking clearly, slowly, and directly. Maintain face-to-face contact whenever possible.

3. Provide privacy for the client.

4. If the client is in bed, raise the head of the bed, use a backrest, or use pillows to have her in an upright sitting position. If the bed is adjustable, adjust bed to a safe level, usually waist high. If the bed is movable, lock bed wheels. If the client is ambulatory, provide a chair.

5. Place the towel under the client's head or around the shoulders.

6. Remove any hairpins, hair ties, and clips.

7. Remove tangles first by dividing hair into small sections. Hold the lock of hair just above the tangle so you do not pull at the scalp. Gently comb or brush through the tangle. If client agrees, you can use a small amount of detangler or leave-in conditioner.

8. After tangles are removed, brush two-inch sections of hair at a time. Gently brush from roots to ends (Fig. 4-55).

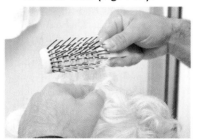

Fig. 4-55. Gently brush hair after tangles are removed.

9. Neatly style hair as client prefers. Avoid childish hairstyles. Each client may prefer different hairstyles. Offer a mirror to the client.

10. Remove the towel and shake excess hair in the wastebasket. Place the soiled towel in the hamper. Store supplies. Clean hair from brush/comb. If you raised an adjustable bed, return it to its lowest position.

11. Wash your hands.

12. Document the procedure and any observations.

Fingernails can harbor bacteria. It is important to keep hands and nails clean to help prevent infection. Nail care should be given when nails are dirty or have jagged edges and whenever it has been assigned. Some agencies do not allow HHAs to cut a client's fingernails or toenails. Poor circulation can lead to infection if skin is accidentally cut while caring for nails. For a diabetic client, such an infection can lead to a severe wound or even amputation. HHAs should follow their agency's policies and the care plan's instructions.

Providing fingernail care

Equipment: orangewood stick, emery board, small basin or bowl, soap, washcloth, 2 towels, lotion, bath thermometer (if available), gloves

1. Wash your hands.

2. Explain the procedure to the client, speaking clearly, slowly, and directly. Maintain face-to-face contact whenever possible.

3. Provide privacy for the client.

4. If the bed is adjustable, adjust bed to a safe working level, usually waist high. If the bed is movable, lock bed wheels.

5. If necessary, remove nail polish with a cotton ball soaked with nail polish remover.

6. Fill the basin halfway with warm water. Test water temperature with the thermometer or against the inside of your wrist to ensure it is safe. Water temperature should be no higher than 105°F. Have the client check the water temperature. Adjust if necessary. Place basin at a comfortable level for the client.

7. Put on gloves.

8. Soak the client's hands and nails in the basin of water. Soak all 10 fingertips for at least five minutes.

9. Remove hands from water. Wash hands with soapy washcloth. Rinse. Pat hands dry with towel, including between fingers. Remove the basin.

10. Place client's hands on the towel. Gently clean under each fingernail with orangewood stick (Fig. 4-56).

11. Wipe orangewood stick on towel after each nail. Wash client's hands again. Dry them thoroughly, especially between fingers.

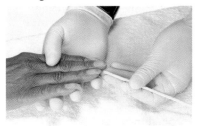

Fig. 4-56. Be gentle when removing dirt from under the nails with an orangewood stick.

12. Shape nails with file or emery board. File in a curve. Finish with nails smooth and free of rough edges.

13. Apply lotion from fingertips to wrists. Remove excess, if any, with a towel.

14. Empty, rinse, and dry the basin. Dispose of the towels in the laundry hamper and store supplies. If you raised an adjustable bed, return it to its lowest position.

15. Remove and discard gloves. Wash your hands.

16. Document procedure and any observations.

Providing foot care

Equipment: basin, bath mat, soap, lotion, washcloth, 2 bath towels, bath thermometer, clean socks, gloves

1. Wash your hands.

2. Explain the procedure to the client, speaking clearly, slowly, and directly. Maintain face-to-face contact whenever possible.

3. Provide privacy for the client.

4. If client is in bed, and the bed is adjustable, adjust bed to a safe working level, usually waist high. If the bed is movable, lock bed wheels.

5. Fill the basin halfway with warm water. Test water temperature with the thermometer or against the inside of your wrist to ensure it is safe. Water temperature should be no higher than 105°F. Have the client check the water temperature. Adjust if necessary.

6. Place basin on a bath mat or bath towel on the floor (if the client is sitting in a chair) or on a towel at the foot of the bed (if the client is in bed). Make sure basin is in a comfortable position for client. Support the foot and ankle throughout the procedure.

7. Put on gloves.

8. Remove client's socks. Completely submerge the client's feet in water. Soak the feet for 10 to 20 minutes. Add warm water to the basin as necessary.

9. Put soap on wet washcloth. Remove one foot from water. Wash entire foot, including

between the toes and around nail beds (Fig. 4-57).

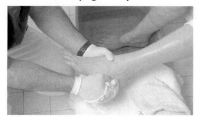

Fig. 4-57. *Soak the client's feet first before washing the entire foot, including the nail beds.*

10. Rinse entire foot, including between the toes.

11. Thoroughly dry entire foot, including between the toes.

12. Repeat steps 9-11 for other foot.

13. Put lotion in one hand and warm the lotion by rubbing hands together. Massage lotion into entire foot (top and bottom), except between the toes. Remove excess, if any, with a towel.

15. Help client to put on clean socks.

16. Empty, rinse, and dry the basin. Dispose of the towels in the laundry hamper and store supplies. If you raised an adjustable bed, return it to its lowest position.

17. Remove and discard gloves. Wash your hands.

18. Document procedure and any observations. Was there any redness, whiteness, or broken or discolored skin or nails? Were there any differences in temperature of the feet?

The HHA should make sure the client wants her to shave him or help him shave. Personal preferences for shaving must be respected. HHAs must wear gloves when shaving clients due to risk of exposure to blood.

Shaving a client

Equipment: razor, basin filled halfway with warm water (if using a safety or disposable razor), shaving cream or soap (if using a safety or disposable razor), 2 towels, washcloth, mirror, after-shave lotion, gloves

1. Wash your hands.

2. Explain the procedure to the client, speaking clearly, slowly, and directly. Maintain face-to-face contact whenever possible.

3. Provide privacy for the client.

4. Place the equipment on a table within reach of the client if he will shave himself. If the client is in bed, raise the head of the bed, use a backrest, or use pillows to have him in an upright sitting position. If the bed is adjustable, adjust bed to a safe level, usually waist high. If the bed is movable, lock bed wheels. If the client wears dentures, be sure they are in place. Place the towel across the client's chest, under his chin.

5. Put on gloves.

Shaving using a safety or disposable razor:

6. Make sure blade is sharp. A dull blade is hard on the skin. Soften the beard with a warm, wet washcloth on the face for a few minutes before shaving. Lather the face with shaving cream or soap and warm water. Warm water and lather make shaving more comfortable.

7. Hold skin taut. Shave in the direction of hair growth. Shave

beard in downward strokes on face and upward strokes on neck (Fig. 4-58). Rinse the blade often in warm water to keep it clean and wet.

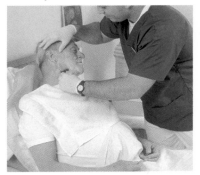

Fig. 4-58. Holding the skin taut, shave in downward strokes on face and upward strokes on neck.

8. When you have finished, wash and rinse the client's face with a warm, wet washcloth. If he is able, let him use the washcloth himself. Use the towel to dry his face. Offer a mirror to the client.

Shaving using an electric razor:

6. Use a small brush to clean the razor. Do not use an electric razor near any water source or when oxygen is in use.

7. Turn on the razor and hold skin taut. Shave with smooth, even movements (Fig. 4-59). Shave beard with back and forth motion in direction of beard growth with foil shaver. Shave beard in circular motion with three-head shaver. Shave the chin and under the chin.

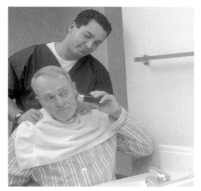

Fig. 4-59. Shave, or have client shave, with smooth, even movements.

8. Offer a mirror to the client.

Final steps:

9. Apply after-shave lotion if the client wants it.

10. Remove the towel. Place the towel and washcloth in the hamper or laundry basket. If you raised an adjustable bed, return it to its lowest position.

11. Clean the equipment and store it. For safety razor, rinse the razor. For disposable razor, dispose of it in a sharps container if available. For electric razor, clean head of razor. Remove whiskers from razor. Recap shaving head and return razor to case.

12. Remove and discard gloves. Wash your hands.

13. Make sure that client and environment are free of loose hairs.

14. Document the procedure and any observations.

Guidelines: Helping a Client Dress and Undress

G   Ask and follow the client's preferences. Let the client choose clothing for the day. Check to see if it is clean, appropriate for the weather, and in good condition.

G   Encourage the client to dress in regular clothes rather than night-clothes. Clothing with elastic waistbands and clothing that is a size larger than normal are easier to put on.

G   Let the client do as much to dress or undress himself as possible. Assistive devices for dressing are available. They help maintain independence. Use them as directed.

G   Provide privacy and never expose more than is needed.

G   Roll or fold socks or stockings down when putting them on. Slip over the toes and foot, then unroll into place.

G   For a female client, make sure bra cups fit over the breasts. A front-fastening bra is easier for clients to fasten by themselves.

G   If a client has a weakened side due to a stroke or injury, that side is called the *affected* or *involved* side. It will be weaker. Never refer to the weaker side as the "bad side" or talk about the "bad" leg or arm. Use the terms *weaker*, *affected*, or *involved* to refer to the affected side.

G Place the weaker arm or leg through the garment first, then help with the stronger arm or leg. When undressing, do the opposite— start with the stronger, or unaffected, side.

Oral Care

Oral care, or care of the mouth, teeth, and gums, is done at least twice each day. Oral care should be done after breakfast and after the last meal or snack of the day. It may also be done before a client eats. Oral care includes brushing teeth, tongue, and gums; flossing teeth; caring for lips; and caring for dentures. Gloves must be worn when giving oral care. HHAs should follow Standard Precautions.

Observing and Reporting: Oral Care

%ʀ Irritation

%ʀ Raised areas

%ʀ Coated or swollen tongue

%ʀ Ulcers, such as canker sores or small, painful, white sores

%ʀ Flaky, white spots

%ʀ Dry, cracked, bleeding, or chapped lips

%ʀ Loose, chipped, broken, or decayed teeth

%ʀ Swollen, irritated, bleeding, or whitish gums

%ʀ Breath that smells bad or fruity

%ʀ Client reports of mouth pain

Providing oral care

Equipment: toothbrush, toothpaste, emesis basin, bath towel, glass of water, lip moisturizer, gloves

1. Wash your hands.

2. Explain the procedure to the client, speaking clearly, slowly, and directly. Maintain face-to-face contact whenever possible.

3. Provide privacy for the client.

4. If the client is in bed, raise the head of the bed, use a backrest, or use pillows to have him in an upright sitting position. If the bed is adjustable, adjust bed to a safe level, usually waist high. If the bed is movable, lock bed wheels.

5. Put on gloves.

6. Place a towel across the client's chest.

7. Remove any dental bridgework or ask your client to do so.

8. Wet toothbrush and put a small amount of toothpaste on it.

9. Clean entire mouth, including tongue and all surfaces of the teeth and gumline. Use gentle strokes. First brush inner, outer, and chewing surfaces of the upper teeth. Then do the

same with the lower teeth. Use short strokes. Brush back and forth. Brush tongue.

10. Give the client water to rinse the mouth. Place emesis basin under the client's chin, with the inward curve under the chin. Have client spit water into emesis basin (Fig. 4-60). Wipe the client's mouth and remove towel.

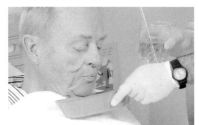

Fig. 4-60. *Rinsing and spitting removes food particles and toothpaste.*

11. Replace any dental bridgework. Apply lip moisturizer if the client desires.

12. Rinse toothbrush and place in proper container. Empty, rinse, and dry basin. Put the soiled towels in the laundry hamper. Store supplies. If you raised an adjustable bed, return it to its lowest position.

13. Remove and discard gloves. Wash your hands.

14. Document the procedure and any observations. Did you observe any mouth ulcers or other broken skin? What was the condition of the mucous membrane? Report any problems with teeth, mouth, tongue, and lips to your supervisor. This includes odor, cracking, sores, bleeding, and any discoloration.

Even though clients who are unconscious cannot eat, breathing through the mouth causes saliva to dry in the mouth. Oral care needs to be performed more frequently to keep the mouth clean and moist. With unconscious clients, HHAs must use as little liquid as possible when giving oral care. Because the person's swallowing reflex is weak, he or she is at risk for aspiration. **Aspiration** is the inhalation of food, fluid, or foreign material into the lungs. Aspiration can cause pneumonia or death. Turning unconscious clients on their sides before giving oral care can also help prevent aspiration. For these clients, only swabs soaked in tiny amounts of fluid should be used to clean the mouth.

Providing oral care for the unconscious client

Equipment: sponge swabs, tongue depressor, emesis basin or small bowl, towel, glass of water, cleaning solution (check the care plan), lip moisturizer, gloves

1. Wash your hands.

2. Explain the procedure to the client, speaking clearly, slowly, and directly. Maintain face-to-face contact whenever possible.

Even clients who are unconscious may be able to hear you. Always speak to them as you would to any client.

3. Provide privacy for the client.

4. If the bed is adjustable, adjust bed to a safe level, usually waist high. If the bed is movable, lock bed wheels.

5. Put on gloves.

6. Turn client on his side or turn his head to the side. Place a towel under his cheek and chin. Place emesis basin or bowl next to the cheek and chin for excess fluid.

7. Hold mouth open with tongue depressor.

8. Dip the sponge swab in cleaning solution. Squeeze out excess solution to prevent aspiration. Wipe teeth, gums, tongue, and inside surfaces of the mouth. Remove debris with the swab. Change swab often. Repeat this step until the mouth is clean (Fig. 4-61).

9. Rinse with clean swab dipped in water. Squeeze swab first to remove excess water.

10. Remove the towel and basin. Pat lips or face dry if needed. Apply lip moisturizer.

11. Empty, rinse, and dry basin. Place the towel in the laundry hamper. Store supplies. If you raised an adjustable bed, return it to its lowest position.

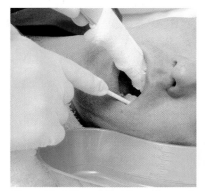

Fig. 4-61. *Wipe all inside surfaces of the mouth to clean the mouth, stimulate the gums, and remove mucus.*

12. Remove and discard gloves. Wash your hands.

13. Document the procedure and any observations. Did you observe any mouth ulcers or other broken skin? What was the condition of the mucous membrane? Report any problems with teeth, mouth, tongue, and lips to your supervisor. This includes odor, cracking, sores, bleeding, and any discoloration.

Flossing the teeth removes plaque and tartar buildup around the gum line and between the teeth. Teeth may be flossed immediately after or before they are brushed, as the client prefers.

Flossing teeth

Equipment: dental floss, glass of water, emesis basin, face towel, gloves

1. Wash your hands.

2. Explain the procedure to the client, speaking clearly, slowly, and directly. Maintain face-to-face contact whenever possible.

3. Provide privacy for the client.

4. If your client is in bed, raise the head of the bed, use a backrest, or use pillows to have him in an upright sitting position. If the bed is adjustable, adjust bed to a safe level, usually waist high. If the bed is movable, lock bed wheels.

5. Put on gloves.

6. Wrap the ends of the floss securely around each index finger (Fig. 4-62).

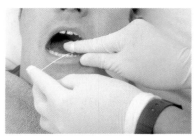

Fig. 4-62. Before beginning, wrap floss securely around each index finger.

7. **Starting with the back teeth, place the floss between teeth and move it down the surface of the tooth using a gentle sawing motion. Continue to the gum line. At the gum line, curve the floss. Slip it gently into the space between the gum and tooth, then go back up, scraping that side of the tooth. Repeat this on the side of the other tooth.**

8. **After every two teeth, unwind floss from your fingers and move it so you are using a clean area. Floss all teeth.**

9. **Occasionally offer water so that the client can rinse debris from the mouth into the basin.**

10. **Offer the client a face towel when done flossing all teeth.**

11. **Discard floss. Discard water and rinse and dry the basin. Put the soiled face towel in the laundry hamper. Store supplies. If you raised an adjustable bed, return it to its lowest position.**

12. **Remove and discard gloves. Wash your hands.**

13. **Document procedure and any observations. Report any problems with teeth, mouth, tongue, and lips to your supervisor. This includes odor, cracking, sores, bleeding, and any discoloration.**

Dentures are artificial teeth. They are expensive, so it is important to take good care of them. Dentures must be handled carefully to avoid breaking or chipping them. If a client's dentures break, he or she cannot eat. HHAs must wear gloves when handling or cleaning dentures. The HHA should notify the supervisor if a client's dentures do not fit properly, are chipped, or are missing. Each person may have his own preference about when and how denture care should be done. The HHA should ask the client how she can assist with denture care. Dentures should be stored in a denture cup filled with solution or clean, moderate temperature water when not in the client's mouth.

Cleaning and storing dentures

Equipment: denture brush or toothbrush, denture cleanser or toothpaste, denture cup, 2 towels, gauze squares, gloves

1. **Wash your hands.**

2. **Explain the procedure to the client, speaking clearly, slowly, and directly. Maintain face-to-face contact whenever possible.**

3. **Provide privacy for the client.**

4. **Put on gloves.**

5. **Line the sink or a basin with one or two towels and partially fill sink with water. The towel and water will prevent the dentures from breaking if they slip from your hands and fall into the sink.**

6. Ask the client to remove the dentures and place them in the denture cup. If the client is unable to remove them, do it yourself. Remove the lower denture first. The lower denture is easier to remove because it floats on the gum line of the lower jaw. Grasp the lower denture with a gauze square (for a good grip) and remove it. Place it in a denture cup filled with moderate temperature water.

7. The upper denture is sealed by suction. Firmly grasp the upper denture with a gauze square and give a slight downward pull to break the suction. Turn it at an angle to take it out of the mouth.

8. Take the denture cup to the sink or basin. Rinse dentures in moderate temperature running water before brushing them. Do not use hot water, or dentures may warp.

9. Apply toothpaste or denture cleanser to brush.

10. Brush dentures on all surfaces (Fig. 4-63). This includes the inner, outer, and chewing surfaces of dentures, as well as the groove that will touch gum surfaces.

11. Rinse all surfaces of dentures under moderate temperature running water. Do not use hot water.

12. Rinse denture cup before placing clean dentures in the cup.

13. Your client may prefer to clean the dentures with a soaking solution. Read the directions on the bottle and prepare the solution. Soak the dentures for the amount of time indicated. Rinse and place in denture cup.

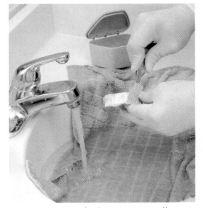

Fig. 4-63. Brush dentures on all surfaces to properly clean them.

14. Store dentures in solution or moderate temperature water to prevent them from warping. Place lid on cup. To avoid accidentally throwing dentures away, always store them in a labeled denture cup when the client is not wearing them. Some clients will want to wear dentures all of the time. They will only remove them for cleaning. If the client wants to continue wearing dentures, return them to him or her. Do not place them in the denture cup.

15. Rinse brush. Dry and return equipment to storage. Drain sink. Put towels in laundry hamper.

16. Remove and discard gloves. Wash your hands.

17. Document procedure and any observations. Report any change in appearance of dentures to the supervisor.

Reinserting dentures

Equipment: denture cup with dentures, denture cream or adhesive, towel, gloves

Ask if the client needs your assistance in inserting dentures.

1. **Wash your hands.**

2. **Explain the procedure to the client, speaking clearly, slowly, and directly. Maintain face-to-face contact whenever possible.**

3. **Provide privacy for the client.**

4. **Position client as you would for brushing teeth (help her into an upright position).**

5. **Put on gloves.**

6. **Apply denture cream or adhesive to the dentures if needed.**

7. **Ask client to open her mouth. Insert the upper denture into the mouth by turning it at an angle. Straighten it and press it onto the upper gum line firmly and evenly (Fig. 4-64).**

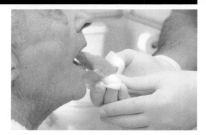

Fig. 4-64. *Press upper denture onto the upper gum line firmly and evenly.*

8. **Place the lower denture on the gum line of the lower jaw and press firmly.**

9. **Offer the client the towel.**

10. **Rinse and store the denture cup. Place the towel in the laundry hamper and store supplies.**

11. **Remove and discard gloves. Wash your hands.**

12. **Document the procedure and any observations.**

Toileting

Clients who are unable to get out of bed to use the toilet may be given a bedpan, a fracture pan, or a urinal. A fracture pan is a bedpan that is flatter than a regular bedpan. It is used for clients who cannot assist with raising their hips onto a regular bedpan. Women will generally use a bedpan for urination and bowel movements. Men will generally use a urinal for urination and a bedpan for bowel movements.

Urine and feces are considered infectious wastes. Wastes should always be discarded in the toilet. HHAs should be careful not to spill or splash the wastes.

HHAs must always wear gloves when handling bedpans, urinals, or basins that contain wastes, including dirty bath water. These containers should be washed thoroughly. After washing these containers, the HHA should remove his gloves and wash his hands. He should put on a new pair of gloves if he is not finished with client care.

Washcloths used to clean perineal areas must be washed in hot water. The HHA should wear gloves when handling these washcloths. Washing them separately is safest. Disposable wipes may or may not be flushable. The package will have this information. If they are not flushable, wipes should be disposed of in a waste container lined with a plastic bag. The HHA should remove and replace the plastic bag frequently to prevent odors.

Assisting client with use of a bedpan

Equipment: bedpan, bedpan cover (newspaper or washable cloth), protective pad, bath blanket, toilet paper, disposable wipes, soap, towel, plastic bag, 2 pairs of gloves, talcum powder (if needed)

1. Wash your hands.

2. Explain the procedure to the client, speaking clearly, slowly, and directly. Maintain face-to-face contact whenever possible.

3. Provide privacy for the client by closing doors and shades and using a covering blanket.

4. If the bed is adjustable, adjust bed to a safe level, usually waist high. Before placing bedpan, lower the head of the bed. If the bed is movable, lock bed wheels.

5. Put on gloves.

6. Warm outside of the bedpan with warm water in the bathroom and cover it when you bring it to the client. Dust the top of the bedpan with talcum powder to prevent it from sticking to the client's skin. Do not use talcum powder if the client has open sores on the buttocks or genitals. Do not use powder if a stool or urine sample is needed. If a stool or urine sample is not needed, place a few sheets of toilet paper in the bedpan to make cleanup easier.

7. Cover the client with the bath blanket and ask him to hold it while you pull down the top covers underneath it. Do not expose more of the client's body than you need to.

8. Place a protective pad under the client's buttocks and hips. To do this, have the client roll toward you. If the client cannot do this, you must turn him toward you. Be sure the client cannot roll off the bed. Move to the empty side of the bed. Place the protective pad on the area where the client will lie on his back. The side of the protective pad nearest the client should be fanfolded (folded several times into pleats) and tucked under the client (Fig. 4-65).

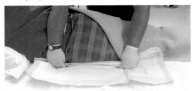

Fig. 4-65. Fanfold the protective pad near the client's back.

Ask the client to roll onto his back, or roll him as you did before. Unfold the rest of the protective pad so it completely covers the area under and around the client's hips (Fig. 4-66).

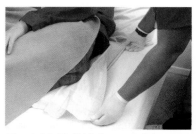

Fig. 4-66. *Unfold the rest of the protective pad so it completely covers area under and around the client's hips.*

9. Ask the client to remove undergarments or help him do so.

10. Place the bedpan near his hips in the correct position. A standard bedpan should be positioned with the wider end aligned with the client's buttocks. A fracture pan should be positioned with handle toward foot of the bed.

11. If client is able, ask him to raise hips by pushing with feet and hands at the count of three (Fig. 4-67). Slide the bedpan under his hips.

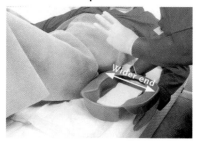

Fig. 4-67. *On the count of three, slide the bedpan under the client's hips. The wider end of bedpan should be aligned with the client's buttocks.*

If the client cannot do this himself, place your arm under the small of his back. Tell him to push with his heels and hands on your signal as you raise his hips (Fig. 4-68).

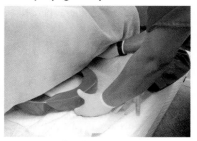

Fig. 4-68. *If a client cannot raise his hips, you can raise his hips while he pushes with his heels and hands.*

If a client cannot help you in any way, keep the bed flat and roll the client away from you. Slip the bedpan under his hips and gently roll the client back onto the bedpan. Keep the bedpan centered underneath.

12. Remove and discard gloves. Wash your hands.

13. Raise the head of the bed. Prop the client into a semi-sitting position using pillows.

14. Make sure the bath blanket is still covering the client. Place toilet paper and disposable wipes within client's reach. Ask client to clean his hands with a wipe when finished if he is able.

15. Place a bell or other way to call you within client's reach. Ask the client to signal when done and explain that you will return when called. Leave the room and close the door.

16. When called by the client, return and put on clean gloves.

17. Lower the head of the bed. Make sure client is still covered.

18. Remove bedpan carefully and cover bedpan.

19. Provide perineal care if help is needed. Wipe female clients from front to back. Dry the perineal area with a towel. Help the client put on undergarment. Cover the client and remove the bath blanket.

20. Wrap the toilet paper and disposable wipes in a plastic bag and discard the bag. Remove and discard protective pad. Place the towel and bath blanket in a hamper.

21. Take bedpan to the bathroom. Empty the bedpan carefully into the toilet unless a specimen is needed or urine is being monitored for intake/output monitoring. Note color, odor, and consistency of contents before flushing. If you notice anything unusual about the stool or urine (for example, the presence of blood), do not discard it. You will need to notify your supervisor.

22. Using a paper towel, turn on the faucet. Rinse the bedpan with cold water and empty it into the toilet. Flush the toilet. Then clean the bedpan with hot, soapy water and store.

23. Remove and discard gloves. Wash your hands.

24. If you raised an adjustable bed, return it to its lowest position.

25. Document the time of the elimination, the contents, and any observations.

Assisting a male client with a urinal

Equipment: urinal, protective pad, disposable wipes, soap, 2 pairs of gloves

1. Wash your hands.

2. Explain the procedure to the client, speaking clearly, slowly, and directly. Maintain face-to-face contact whenever possible.

3. Provide privacy for the client by closing doors and shades and using a covering blanket.

4. If the bed is adjustable, adjust bed to a safe level, usually waist high. If the bed is movable, lock bed wheels.

5. Put on gloves.

6. Place a protective pad under the client's buttocks and hips, as in earlier procedure.

7. Hand the urinal to the client. If the client is not able to help himself, place the urinal between his legs and position the penis inside the urinal (Fig. 4-69). Replace covers.

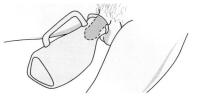

Fig. 4-69. Position the penis inside the urinal if the client cannot do it himself.

8. Remove and discard gloves. Wash your hands.

9. Place disposable wipes within client's reach. Ask the client to clean his hands with a wipe when finished if he is able. Give the client a bell or another way to call you. Ask the client to signal when done and explain that you will return

when called. Leave the room and close the door.

10. When called by the client, return and put on clean gloves.

11. Discard disposable wipes.

12. Remove the urinal or have client hand it to you. Empty contents into toilet unless a specimen is needed or the client's urine is being measured for intake/output monitoring. Note color, odor, and qualities (for example, cloudiness) of contents before flushing.

13. Using a paper towel, turn on the faucet. Rinse the urinal with cold water and empty it into the toilet. Flush the toilet. Store the urinal.

14. Remove and discard gloves. Wash your hands.

15. If you raised an adjustable bed, return it to its lowest position.

16. Document the time, the amount of urine (if monitoring intake and output), and any observations.

Some clients are able to get out of bed, but may still need help walking to the bathroom and using the toilet. Others who are able to get out of bed but cannot walk to the bathroom may use a portable commode, or bedside commode (BSC). A portable commode is a chair with a toilet seat and a removable container underneath (Fig. 4-70).

Toilets can be fitted with raised seats to make it easier for clients to get up and down. Hand rails can also be installed next to the toilet. The HHA should report to the supervisor if these assistive devices are needed. When clients need assistance to get to the bathroom or use the commode, the HHA should offer to help often. This can avoid accidents and embarrassment.

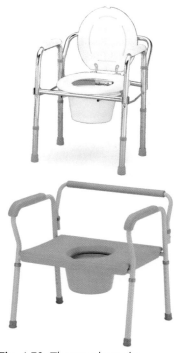

Fig. 4-70. *The top photo shows a regular portable, or bedside, commode, and the bottom photo shows a bariatric portable commode, which can be used for people who are overweight or obese.* (PHOTOS COURTESY OF NOVA MEDICAL PRODUCTS, WWW.NOVAMEDICALPRODUCTS.COM)

Assisting a client to use a portable commode or toilet

Equipment: portable commode with basin, toilet paper, disposable wipes, towel, 3 pairs of gloves

1. Wash your hands.

2. Explain the procedure to the client, speaking clearly, slowly, and directly. Maintain face-to-face contact whenever possible.

3. Provide privacy for the client by closing doors and shades and using a covering blanket.

4. If the bed is movable, lock bed wheels. Make sure client is wearing nonskid shoes and that the laces are tied. Help client out of bed and to the portable commode or bathroom.

5. Put on gloves.

6. If needed, help client remove clothing and sit comfortably on toilet seat. Put toilet paper and disposable wipes within reach. Ask client to clean his hands with a wipe when finished if he is able.

7. Remove and discard gloves. Wash your hands.

8. Provide privacy. Give the client a bell or another way to call you. Leave the room and close the door. Do not go too far away in case you are needed soon.

9. When called by the client, return and put on clean gloves.

Give perineal care if help is needed. Wipe female clients from front to back. Dry the perineal area with a towel. Help client to put on clothing.

10. Place the towel in a hamper or bag. Discard disposable supplies.

11. Remove and discard gloves. Wash your hands.

12. Help the client back to bed.

13. Put on clean gloves.

14. Remove waste container if client used portable commode. Empty it into the toilet unless a specimen is needed or the client's urine is being measured for intake/output monitoring. Note color, odor, and consistency of contents before flushing.

15. Using a paper towel, turn on the faucet. Rinse the container with cold water and empty it into the toilet. Flush the toilet. Then clean the container with hot, soapy water and store.

16. Remove and discard gloves. Wash your hands.

17. Make sure bed is in its lowest position.

18. Document the procedure and any observations.

Vital Signs

Home health aides monitor, document, and report clients' vital signs. Vital signs are important. They show how well the vital organs of the body, such as the heart and lungs, are working. They consist of the following:

- Measuring the body temperature

- Counting the pulse
- Counting the rate of respirations
- Measuring the blood pressure
- Observing and reporting the level of pain

Watching for changes in vital signs is very important. Changes can indicate that a client's condition is worsening. An HHA should always notify the supervisor if

- The client has a fever (temperature is above average for the client or outside the normal range)
- The client has a respiratory or pulse rate that is too rapid or too slow
- The client's blood pressure changes
- The client's pain is worse or is not relieved by pain management

Ranges for Adult Vital Signs		
Temp. Site	**Fahrenheit**	**Celsius**
Mouth (oral)	97.6°–99.6°	36.5°–37.5°
Rectum (rectal)	98.6°–100.6°	37.0°–38.1°
Armpit (axillary)	96.6°–98.6°	36.0°–37.0°
Ear (tympanic)	96.6°–99.7°	35.8°–37.6°
Temporal Artery	97.2°–100.1°	36.2°–37.8°
Normal Pulse Rate: 60–100 beats per minute		
Normal Respiratory Rate: 12–20 respirations per minute		
Blood Pressure		
Normal:	Systolic 100–139 Diastolic 60–89	
Low:	Below 100/60	
High:	140/90 or above	

Temperature

Body temperature is normally very close to 98.6°F (Fahrenheit) or 37°C (Celsius). Body temperature is a balance between the heat created by the body and the heat lost to the environment. Many factors affect body temperature: age, illness, stress, environment, exercise, and the circadian rhythm can all cause changes in body temperature. The circadian rhythm is the 24-hour day-night cycle. Increases in body temperature may indicate an infection or disease. Average temperature readings change throughout the day. People tend to have lower temperatures in the morning. There are different sites for measuring body temperature:

- The mouth (oral)
- The rectum (rectal)
- The armpit (axillary)
- The ear (tympanic)
- The temporal artery (the artery under the skin of the forehead)

There are several types of thermometers, including the following:

- Mercury-free (Fig. 4-71)
- Digital (Fig. 4-72)
- Electronic (Fig. 4-73)
- Disposable (Fig. 4-74)
- Tympanic (Fig. 4-75)
- Temporal artery (Fig. 4-76)

There is a range of normal temperatures. Some people's temperatures normally run low. Others run slightly higher, even in good health. Normal temperature readings also vary by the method used to take the temperature. A rectal temperature is generally considered to be the most accurate. However, taking a rectal temperature on an uncooperative person, such as a client with dementia, can be dangerous. An axillary temperature is considered the least accurate.

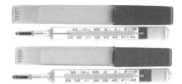

Fig. 4-71. *A mercury-free oral thermometer and a mercury-free rectal thermometer. Oral thermometers are usually green or blue; rectal thermometers are usually red.* (PHOTOS COURTESY OF RG MEDICAL DIAGNOSTICS OF WIXOM, MI, RGMD.COM)

Fig. 4-72. *A digital thermometer.*

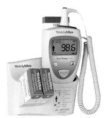

Fig. 4-73. *An electronic thermometer.* (PHOTO COURTESY OF WELCH ALLYN, WWW.WELCHALLYN.COM, 800-535-6663)

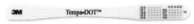

Fig. 4-74. *A disposable thermometer.*

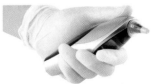

Fig. 4-75. *A tympanic thermometer.*

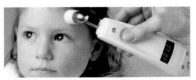

Fig. 4-76. *A temporal artery thermometer.* (PHOTO COURTESY OF EXERGEN CORPORATION, 800-422-3006, WWW.EXERGEN.COM)

Mercury Glass Thermometers

Using mercury glass or glass bulb thermometers to take oral, rectal, or axillary temperatures is no longer common because mercury is a dangerous, toxic substance. In fact, many states have passed laws banning the sale of mercury thermometers. If a client still uses a mercury glass thermometer, the HHA should check with her supervisor about replacing it with a mercury-free thermometer.

Measuring and recording oral temperature

Do not take an oral temperature on a client who has smoked, had food or fluids, chewed gum, or exercised in the last 10 to 20 minutes.

Equipment: clean mercury-free, digital, or electronic thermometer, gloves, disposable sheath/cover for thermometer, tissues, pen and paper

1. Wash your hands.

2. Explain the procedure to the client, speaking clearly, slowly, and directly. Maintain face-to-face contact whenever possible.

3. Provide privacy for the client.

4. Put on gloves.

5. *Mercury-free thermometer*: Hold the thermometer by the stem. Before inserting it in the client's mouth, shake thermometer down to below the lowest number (at least below 96°F or 35°C). To shake the thermometer down, hold it at the side opposite the bulb with the thumb and two fingers. With a snapping motion of the wrist, shake the thermometer (Fig. 4-77). Stand away from furniture and walls while doing so.

   Digital thermometer: Put on the disposable sheath. Turn on thermometer and wait until *ready* sign appears.

Electronic thermometer: Remove the probe from base unit. Put on probe cover.

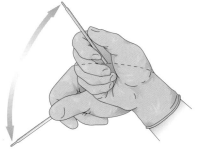

Fig. 4-77. *Shake thermometer down to below the lowest number before inserting in a client's mouth.*

6. *Mercury-free thermometer*: Put on disposable sheath if available. Insert bulb end of the thermometer into client's mouth, under tongue and to one side (Fig. 4-78).

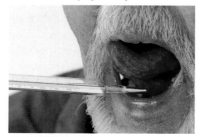

Fig. 4-78. *Insert thermometer under the client's tongue and to one side.*

Digital thermometer: Insert the end of digital thermometer into client's mouth, under tongue and to one side.

Electronic thermometer: Insert the end of electronic thermometer into client's mouth, under tongue and to one side.

7. *For all thermometers*: Tell the client to hold the thermometer in his mouth with lips closed. Assist as necessary. Client should breathe through his nose. Ask the client not to bite down or to talk.

   Mercury-free thermometer: Leave the thermometer in place for at least three minutes.

   Digital thermometer: Leave in place until thermometer blinks or beeps.

   Electronic thermometer: Leave in place until you hear a tone or see a flashing or steady light.

8. *Mercury-free thermometer*: Remove the thermometer. Wipe with a tissue from stem to bulb or remove sheath. Dispose of the tissue or sheath. Hold the thermometer at eye level. Rotate until line appears, roll-

ing the thermometer between your thumb and forefinger. Read the temperature. Remember the temperature reading.

Digital thermometer: Remove the thermometer. Read temperature on display screen. Remember the temperature reading.

Electronic thermometer: Read the temperature on the display screen. Remember the temperature reading. Remove the probe from the mouth.

9. *Mercury-free thermometer*: Clean thermometer with soap and water. Rinse with clean water and dry. Return it to case.

   Digital thermometer: Using a tissue, remove and dispose of sheath. Replace the thermometer in case.

   Electronic thermometer: Press the eject button to discard the cover. Return the probe to the holder.

10. Remove and discard gloves.

11. Wash your hands.

12. Immediately record the temperature, date, time, and method used (oral).

HHAs must always explain what they will do before measuring a rectal temperature. The HHA should ask the client to hold still and reassure him that the procedure will only take a few minutes. The HHA should hold onto the thermometer at all times while taking a rectal temperature.

Measuring and recording rectal temperature

Equipment: clean rectal mercury-free, digital, or electronic thermometer, lubricant, gloves, tissue, disposable sheath/cover, pen and paper

1. Wash your hands.

2. Explain the procedure to the client, speaking clearly, slowly,

and directly. Maintain face-to-face contact whenever possible.

3. Provide privacy for the client.

4. If the bed is adjustable, adjust bed to a safe level, usually waist high. If the bed is movable, lock bed wheels.

5. Assist the client to a left-lying (Sims') position.

6. Fold back the linens to expose only the rectal area.

7. Put on gloves.

8. *Mercury-free thermometer:* Hold thermometer by stem. Shake the thermometer down to below the lowest number.

   Digital thermometer: Put on the disposable sheath. Turn on thermometer and wait until *ready* sign appears.

   Electronic thermometer: Remove the probe from base unit. Put on probe cover.

9. Apply a small amount of lubricant to tip of bulb or probe cover.

10. Separate the buttocks. Gently insert thermometer into rectum 1/2 to 1 inch. Stop if you meet resistance. Do not force the thermometer in (Fig. 4-79).

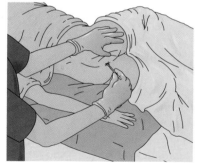

Fig. 4-79. Gently insert a rectal thermometer one-half to one inch into the rectum. Do not force it into the rectum.

11. Replace the sheet over buttocks. Hold on to the thermometer at all times.

12. *Mercury-free thermometer:* Hold thermometer in place for at least three minutes.

    Digital thermometer: Hold thermometer in place until thermometer blinks or beeps.

    Electronic thermometer: Leave in place until you hear a tone or see a flashing or steady light.

13. Gently remove the thermometer. Wipe with tissue from stem to bulb or remove sheath. Discard tissue or sheath.

14. Read the thermometer at eye level as you would for an oral temperature. Remember the temperature reading.

15. *Mercury-free thermometer:* Clean thermometer with soap and water. Rinse with clean water and dry. Return it to case.

    Digital thermometer: Clean thermometer according to policy and replace it in the case.

    Electronic thermometer: Press the eject button to discard the cover. Return the probe to the holder.

16. Remove and discard gloves.

17. Wash your hands.

18. Assist the client to a comfortable position.

19. Immediately record the temperature, date, time, and method used (rectal).

When measuring a tympanic temperature, the HHA should tell the client that she will be placing a thermometer in the ear canal. She should reassure the client that this is painless. The short tip of the thermometer will only go into the ear one-quarter to one-half inch.

Measuring and recording tympanic temperature

Equipment: tympanic thermometer, gloves, disposable sheath/cover, pen and paper

1. Wash your hands.

2. Explain the procedure to the client, speaking clearly, slowly, and directly. Maintain face-to-face contact whenever possible.

3. Provide privacy for the client.

4. Put on gloves.

5. Put a disposable sheath over earpiece of the thermometer.

6. Position the client's head so that the ear is in front of you. Straighten the ear canal by pulling up and back on the outside edge of the ear for an adult (Fig. 4-80). Pull straight back for infants and children. Insert the covered probe into the ear canal. Press the button.

7. Hold thermometer in place either for one second or until thermometer blinks or beeps.

8. Read temperature. Remember the temperature reading.

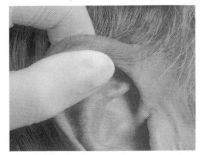

Fig. 4-80. *Straighten the ear canal by pulling up and back on the outside edge of the ear.*

9. Dispose of sheath. Return the thermometer to storage or to the battery charger if thermometer is rechargeable.

10. Remove and discard gloves.

11. Wash your hands.

12. Immediately record the temperature, date, time, and method used (tympanic).

Measuring and recording axillary temperature

Equipment: clean mercury-free, digital, or electronic thermometer, gloves, tissues, disposable sheath/cover, pen and paper

1. Wash your hands.

2. Explain the procedure to the client, speaking clearly, slowly, and directly. Maintain face-to-face contact whenever possible.

3. Provide privacy for the client.

4. Put on gloves.

5. Remove client's arm from sleeve of gown or shirt to allow skin contact with the end of the thermometer. Wipe axillary area

with tissues before placing the thermometer.

6. *Mercury-free thermometer*: Hold the thermometer by the stem. Shake the thermometer down to below the lowest number.

   Digital thermometer: Put on the disposable sheath. Turn on thermometer and wait until *ready* sign appears.

   Electronic thermometer: Remove the probe from base unit. Put on probe cover.

7. Position thermometer (bulb end for mercury-free) in center

of the armpit. Fold client's arm over his chest.

8. *Mercury-free thermometer:* Hold the thermometer in place, with the arm close against the side, for eight to 10 minutes (Fig. 4-81).

   Digital thermometer: Leave in place until thermometer blinks or beeps.

   Electronic thermometer: Leave in place until you hear a tone or see a flashing or steady light.

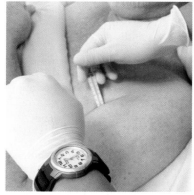

Fig. 4-81. *After inserting the thermometer, fold the client's arm over his chest and hold it in place for eight to 10 minutes.*

9. *Mercury-free thermometer:* Remove the thermometer. Wipe with a tissue from stem to bulb or remove sheath. Dispose of the tissue or sheath. Read the thermometer at eye level as you would for an oral temperature. Remember the temperature reading.

   Digital thermometer: Remove the thermometer. Read temperature on display screen. Remember the temperature reading.

   Electronic thermometer: Read the temperature on the display screen. Remember the temperature reading. Remove the probe.

10. *Mercury-free thermometer:* Clean thermometer with soap and water. Rinse with clean water and dry. Return it to case.

    Digital thermometer: Using a tissue, remove and dispose of sheath. Replace the thermometer in case.

    Electronic thermometer: Press the eject button to discard the cover. Return the probe to the holder.

11. Remove and discard gloves.

12. Wash your hands.

13. Immediately record the temperature, date, time, and method used (axillary).

Pulse

The pulse is the number of times a person's heart beats per minute. The beat that is felt at certain pulse points in the body represents the wave of blood moving through the artery. The most common site for checking the pulse is on the inside of the wrist, where the radial artery runs just beneath the skin. This is called the *radial pulse*. The *brachial pulse* is the pulse inside the elbow, about one to one-and-a-half inches above the elbow. The radial and brachial pulse are involved in taking blood pressure. Blood pressure is explained later in this chapter.

For adults, the normal pulse rate is 60 to 100 beats per minute. Small children have faster pulses, in the range of 100 to 120 beats per minute. A newborn baby's pulse may be as high as 120 to 140 beats per minute. Many things can affect the pulse rate, including exercise, fear, anger, anxiety, heat, infection, medications, and pain. A high or low rate does not necessarily indicate disease. However, sometimes the pulse rate can signal that illness exists. For example, a rapid pulse may result from fever, dehydration, or heart failure. A slow or weak pulse may indicate infection.

The apical pulse is heard by listening directly over the heart with a stethoscope. A stethoscope is an instrument designed to listen to sounds within the body, such as the heart beating or air moving through the lungs. This is often the easiest method for measuring the pulse in infants and small children because their pulse points are harder to find. For adult clients, the apical pulse may be taken when the person has heart disease or takes medication that affects the heart. It may also be taken if clients have a weak radial pulse or an irregular pulse.

Measuring and recording apical pulse

Equipment: stethoscope, alcohol wipes, watch with second hand, pen and paper

1. Wash your hands.

2. Explain the procedure to the client, speaking clearly, slowly, and directly. Maintain face-to-face contact whenever possible.

3. Provide privacy for the client.

4. Before using the stethoscope, wipe the diaphragm and earpieces with alcohol wipes.

5. Fit the earpieces of the stethoscope snugly in your ears. Place the flat metal diaphragm on the left side of the chest, just below the nipple. Listen for the heartbeat.

6. Use the second hand of your watch. Count the heartbeats for one minute (Fig. 4-82). Each lubdub that you hear is counted as one beat. A normal heartbeat is rhythmical. Leave the stethoscope in place to count respirations.

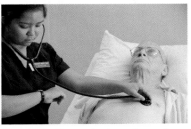

Fig. 4-82. Count the heartbeats for one full minute to measure the apical pulse.

7. Record the pulse rate, date, time, and method used (apical). Note any irregularities in the rhythm.

8. Clean earpieces and diaphragm of stethoscope with alcohol wipes. Store stethoscope.

9. Wash your hands.

Respirations

Respiration is the process of breathing air into the lungs, or inspiration, and exhaling air out of the lungs, or expiration. Each respiration consists of an inspiration and an expiration. The chest rises during inspiration and falls during expiration.

The normal respiration rate for adults ranges from 12 to 20 breaths per minute. Infants and children have a faster respiratory rate; infants normally breathe at a rate of 30 to 40 respirations per minute. People may breathe more quickly if they know they are being observed. Because of this, respirations should be counted immediately after taking the pulse. The HHA should keep her fingers on the client's wrist or on the stethoscope over the heart. She should not make it obvious that she is observing the client's breathing.

Measuring and recording radial pulse and counting and recording respirations

Equipment: watch with a second hand, pen and paper

1. Wash your hands.

2. Explain the procedure to the client, speaking clearly, slowly, and directly. Maintain face-to-face contact whenever possible.

3. Provide privacy for the client.

4. Place fingertips on the thumb side of client's wrist to locate radial pulse (Fig. 4-83).

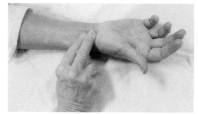

Fig. 4-83. *Measure the radial pulse by placing fingertips on the thumb side of the wrist.*

5. Count the beats for one full minute.

6. Keeping your fingertips on the client's wrist, count respirations for one full minute. Observe for the pattern and character of the client's breathing. Normal breathing is smooth and quiet. If you see signs of difficult, shallow, or noisy breathing, such as wheezing, report it to your supervisor.

7. Record the pulse rate, date, time, and method used (radial). Record the respiratory rate and the pattern or character of breathing. Notify your supervisor if the pulse is less than 60 beats per minute, over 100 beats per minute, or if the rhythm is irregular.

8. Wash your hands.

Blood Pressure

Blood pressure is an important measure of health. Blood pressure is measured in millimeters of mercury (mmHg). The measurement shows how well the heart is working. There are two parts of blood pressure, the systolic measurement and diastolic measurement.

In the **systolic** phase, the heart is at work, contracting and pushing the blood from the left ventricle of the heart. The reading shows the pressure on the walls of arteries as blood is pumped through the body. The normal range for systolic blood pressure is 100 to 119 mmHg.

The second measurement reflects the **diastolic** phase—when the heart relaxes. The diastolic measurement is always lower than the systolic measurement. It shows the pressure in the arteries when the heart is at rest. The normal range for adults is 60 to 79 mmHg.

If blood pressure is between 120/80 mmHg and 139/89 mmHg, it is called *prehypertension*. This means that the person does not have high blood pressure now, but is likely to develop it in the future.

People with high blood pressure, or hypertension, have elevated systolic and/or diastolic blood pressures. A blood pressure level of 140/90 mmHg or higher is considered high. The supervisor should be notified if a client's blood pressure is 140/90 or above.

Many factors can increase blood pressure. These include aging, exercise, physical or emotional stress, pain, medications, and the volume of blood in circulation.

Blood pressure is measured with a stethoscope and a blood pressure cuff, or sphygmomanometer. It is important to use a cuff that is the correct size when measuring blood pressure.

Measuring and recording blood pressure (one-step method)

Equipment: sphygmomanometer (blood pressure cuff), stethoscope, alcohol wipes, pen and paper

1. Wash your hands.

2. Explain the procedure to the client, speaking clearly, slowly, and directly. Maintain face-to-face contact whenever possible.

3. Provide privacy for the client.

4. Before using the stethoscope, wipe the diaphragm and earpieces with alcohol wipes.

5. Ask the client to roll up his sleeve so that the upper arm is exposed. Do not measure blood pressure over clothing.

6. Position the client's arm with the palm up. The arm should be level with the heart.

7. With the valve open, squeeze the cuff to make sure it is completely deflated.

8. Place the blood pressure cuff snugly on client's upper arm. The center of the cuff with the sensor/arrow is placed over the brachial artery (1–1½ inches above the elbow, toward inside of elbow) (Fig. 4-84).

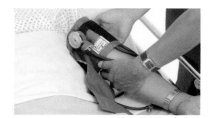

Fig. 4-84. *Place the center of the cuff over the brachial artery.*

9. Locate the brachial pulse with your fingertips.

10. Place earpieces of stethoscope in your ears.

11. Place the diaphragm of the stethoscope over brachial artery.

12. Close the valve (clockwise) until it stops. Do not over-tighten it (Fig. 4-85).

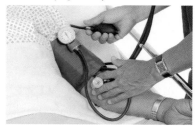

Fig. 4-85. *Close the valve by turning it clockwise. Do not over-tighten it.*

13. Inflate cuff to between 160 mmHg to 180 mmHg. If a beat is heard immediately upon cuff

deflation, completely deflate cuff. Reinflate cuff to no more than 200 mmHg.

14. Open the valve slightly with thumb and index finger. Deflate cuff slowly.

15. Watch gauge. Listen for sound of the pulse.

16. Remember the reading at which the first pulse sound is heard. This is the systolic pressure.

17. Continue listening for a change or muffling of pulse sound. The point of a change or the point at which the sound disappears is the diastolic pressure. Remember this reading.

18. Open the valve. Deflate cuff completely. Remove cuff.

19. Wash your hands.

20. Record both the systolic and diastolic pressures. Record the numbers like a fraction, with the systolic reading on top and the diastolic reading on the bottom (for example: 120/80). Note which arm was used. Use *RA* for right arm and *LA* for left arm.

21. Wipe diaphragm and earpieces of stethoscope with alcohol wipes. Store equipment.

22. Wash your hands.

Pain

HHAs must observe and report clients' pain carefully. Pain is uncomfortable. It can quickly drain energy and hope. It is also a personal (subjective) experience. This means it is different for each person. HHAs play an important role in pain monitoring and prevention. Pain is not a normal part of aging. HHAs must treat clients' complaints of pain seriously. If a client complains of pain, the HHA should ask these questions and then immediately report the information to his supervisor:

• Where is the pain?

- When did the pain start?
- Is the pain mild, moderate or severe? To help find out, the HHA can ask the client to rate the pain on a scale of 0 to 10, with 0 being no pain and 10 being the worst pain.
- Can you describe the pain? The HHA should use the client's words when reporting to the supervisor.
- What were you doing before the pain started?
- How long does the pain last, and how often does it occur?
- What makes the pain better? What makes the pain worse?

To help reduce pain, the HHA should do the following:
- Report complaints of pain or unrelieved pain promptly to the supervisor.
- Gently position the body in proper alignment. Use pillows for support. Assist in frequent changes of position if the client desires it.
- Give back rubs.
- Ask if the client would like to take a warm bath or shower.
- Help the client to the bathroom or offer the bedpan or urinal.
- Encourage slow, deep breathing.
- Provide a calm and quiet environment. Soft music may distract the client.
- Remind the client when it is time to take pain medication.
- Be patient, caring, gentle, and sympathetic.

Pain management is a very important part of palliative care. **Palliative care** is a type of care that focuses on relieving the pain and stress of a serious illness to improve the patient's quality of life. Palliative care is provided as part of hospice care, but may also be given to people who do not have a terminal illness.

Height and Weight

HHAs may measure clients' weight and height as part of care. Height is checked less often than weight. Weight changes can be signs of illness. They can also affect the medication doses a client needs. For these reasons, any weight loss or gain, no matter how small, should be reported.

Measuring and recording weight of an ambulatory client

Equipment: bathroom scale or standing/upright scale, pen and paper

1. Wash your hands.
2. Explain the procedure to the client, speaking clearly, slowly, and directly. Maintain face-to-face contact whenever possible.
3. Provide privacy for the client.
4. If using a bathroom scale, set the scale on a hard surface (not on carpet) in a place the client can get to easily.

5. Make sure the client is wearing nonskid shoes that are fastened before walking to scale.

6. Start with the scale balanced at zero before weighing the client.

7. Help client to step onto the center of the scale. Be sure she is not holding, touching, or leaning against anything. This interferes with weight measurement. Do not force someone to let go. If you are unable to obtain a weight, notify your supervisor.

7. Determine the client's weight. *Using a bathroom scale*: read the weight on the display screen or when the dial has stopped moving. *Using a*

standing scale: this is done by balancing the scale. Move the small and large weight indicators until the bar balances. Read the two numbers shown (on the small and large weight indicators) when the bar is balanced. Add these two numbers together. This is the client's weight.

8. Help the client to safely step off scale before recording weight.

9. Record the client's weight. Report any changes in client's weight to your supervisor.

10. Store the scale if it was moved.

11. Wash your hands.

Measuring and recording height of a client

Some clients will be unable to get out of bed. If so, height can be measured using a tape measure.

Equipment: tape measure, pencil, pen and paper

1. Wash your hands.

2. Explain the procedure to the client, speaking clearly, slowly, and directly. Maintain face-to-face contact whenever possible.

3. Provide privacy for the client.

4. Position the client lying straight in bed, flat on his back with arms at his sides. Be sure the bed sheet is smooth underneath the client.

5. Make a pencil mark on the sheet at the top of the head.

6. Make another mark at the client's heel (Fig. 4-86).

7. With the tape measure, measure the distance between the marks.

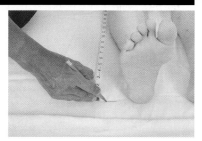

Fig. 4-86. Make marks on the sheet at the client's head and feet.

8. Record the height.

9. Store equipment.

10. Wash your hands.

For clients who can get out of bed, you will measure height while they stand against a wall.

Equipment: tape measure, pencil, pen and paper

1. Wash your hands.

2. Explain the procedure to the client, speaking clearly, slowly,

and directly. Maintain face-to-face contact whenever possible.

3. Provide privacy for the client.

4. Have the client stand with his back to the wall, with his arms at his sides and without shoes. A hard floor is better than carpet.

5. Make a pencil mark on the wall at the top of the client's head.

6. Determine the client's height. Ask client to step away. Use the tape measure to measure the distance between the pencil mark and the floor.

7. Record the height.

8. Store equipment.

9. Wash your hands.

For clients who can get out of bed, you can also measure height using a standing scale.

Equipment: standing scale, pen and paper

1. Wash your hands.

2. Explain the procedure to the client, speaking clearly, slowly, and directly. Maintain face-to-face contact whenever possible.

3. Provide privacy for the client.

4. Help the client to step onto scale, facing away from the scale.

5. Ask the client to stand up straight if possible. Help as needed. Pull up measuring rod from back of the scale and gently lower the rod until it rests flat on the client's head.

6. Determine the client's height.

7. Assist the client to step off scale before recording height.

8. Record the height.

9. Wash your hands.

Special Procedures

Intake and Output (I&O)

The fluid a person consumes is called **intake**, or input. Fluid comes in the form of liquids that a person drinks. It is also found in semi-liquid foods like gelatin, soup, ice cream, pudding, and yogurt. All fluid taken in each day cannot remain in the body. It must be eliminated as **output**. Output includes urine, feces (including diarrhea), and vomitus. It also includes perspiration, moisture in the air that a person exhales, and wound drainage.

Fluid balance is maintaining equal input and output, or taking in and eliminating equal amounts of fluid. Most people do this naturally. But some clients must have their intake and output, or I&O, monitored and recorded. To do this, the HHA will need to measure and record all fluids the client takes by mouth, as well as all urine and vomitus produced. This is recorded on an Intake/Output (I&O) sheet. It can also be recorded on regular paper if no form is provided.

Conversions

One milliliter (mL) is a unit of measure equal to one cubic centimeter (cc). HHAs should follow their agency's policies on whether to document using mL or cc.

1 teaspoon = 5 mL

1 tablespoon = 15 mL

2 tablespoons = 30 mL or 1 oz

1 oz = 30 mL or 30 cc

2 oz = 60 mL

3 oz = 90 mL

4 oz = 120 mL

5 oz = 150 mL

6 oz = 180 mL

7 oz = 210 mL

8 oz = 240 mL

¼ cup = 2 oz = 60 mL

½ cup = 4 oz = 120 mL

1 cup = 8 oz = 240 mL

Measuring and recording intake and output

Equipment: I&O sheet, graduate (measuring container), pen and paper

Measure intake first.

1. Wash your hands.

2. Explain the procedure to the client, speaking clearly, slowly, and directly. Maintain face-to-face contact whenever possible.

3. Provide privacy for the client.

4. Using the graduate, measure how much fluid a client is served. Note the amount on paper, not in the visit notes.

5. When client has finished a meal or snack, measure any leftover fluids. Note this amount on paper.

6. Subtract the leftover amount from the amount served. If you have measured in ounces, convert to milliliters (mL) by multiplying by 30.

7. Document the amount of fluid consumed (in mL) in the input column on I&O form or in the visit notes. Record the time and what fluid was taken. Report anything unusual that was observed, such as the client refusing to drink, drinking very little, feeling nauseated, etc.

8. Wash your hands.

Measuring output is the other half of monitoring fluid balance.

Equipment: I&O sheet, graduate, gloves, pen and paper

1. Wash your hands.

2. Put on gloves before handling a bedpan or urinal.

3. Pour the contents of the bedpan or urinal into graduate. Do not spill or splash any of the urine.

4. Place graduate on a flat surface. Measure the amount of urine at eye level. Note the amount on paper, converting to mL if necessary.

5. After measuring urine, empty graduate into toilet without splashing.

6. Rinse graduate and pour rinse water into the toilet. Flush the toilet. Clean the graduate and bedpan or urinal and store.

7. Remove and discard gloves.

8. Wash your hands before recording output.

9. Document the time and amount of urine in output column on sheet. For example: 1545 hours, 200 mL urine. To measure vomitus, pour from basin into measuring container, then discard in the toilet. If client vomits on the bed or floor, estimate the amount. Document emesis and amount on the I&O sheet.

Emesis, or vomiting, must be documented. It can be a sign of serious illness or injury or it can be a reaction to medication. Some clients, such as those with cancer undergoing chemotherapy, may vomit frequently as a result of treatment. Because an HHA may not know when a client is going to vomit, she may not have time to explain what she will do and assemble supplies ahead of time. The HHA should talk to the client soothingly as she helps him clean up. She should tell him what she is doing to help him.

Observing, reporting and documenting emesis

1. Put on gloves when client has vomited.

2. Make sure the head is up or turned to one side. Place an emesis basin under the chin. Remove it when vomiting has stopped.

3. Remove soiled linens or clothes. Set aside for laundering. Replace with fresh linens or clothes.

4. If client's intake and output (I&O) is being monitored, measure and note amount of vomitus.

5. Flush vomit down the toilet. Wash, dry, and store basin.

6. Remove and discard gloves.

7. Wash your hands.

8. Put on fresh gloves.

9. Provide comfort to client. Wipe face and mouth, position comfortably, and offer a drink of water (Fig. 4-87). Provide oral care. It helps gets rid of the taste of vomit in the mouth.

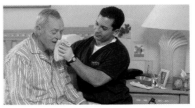

Fig. 4-87. Be calm and comforting when helping a client who has vomited.

10. Launder soiled linens and clothes promptly in hot water.

11. Remove and discard gloves.

12. Wash your hands again.

13. Document time, amount, color, odor, and consistency of vomitus. Look for vomit that is red, has blood in it, or looks like wet coffee grounds, or if medication/pills are in vomit.

14. Report to your supervisor immediately and get instructions for diet.

Catheter Care

A **catheter** is a thin tube inserted into the body that is used to drain or inject fluids. A urinary catheter is used to drain urine from the bladder. A straight catheter does not remain inside a person. It is removed immediately after urine is drained. An indwelling catheter remains inside the bladder for a period of time. The urine drains into a bag. An external, or condom, catheter has an attachment on the end that fits onto the penis. The attachment is fastened with special tape. Urine drains through the catheter into the tubing, then into the drainage bag. The external catheter is changed daily or as needed.

Guidelines: Urinary Catheters

G   Make sure the drainage bag is always lower than the hips or bladder.

G   Keep the drainage bag off the floor.

G   Keep the tubing as straight as possible. It should not be kinked.

G   Keep the genital area clean to prevent infection. Because the catheter goes all the way into the bladder, bacteria can enter the bladder more easily. Daily care of the genital area is especially important.

G   To promote the client's dignity, keep the drainage bag covered.

Observing and Reporting: Catheter Care

%ʀ   Blood in the urine or urine that looks unusual in any way

%ʀ   Catheter bag does not fill after several hours

%ʀ   Catheter bag fills suddenly

%ʀ   Catheter is not in place

%ʀ   Urine leaks from the catheter

%ʀ   Client reports pain or pressure

%ʀ   Odor is present

Providing catheter care

Equipment: bath blanket, protective pad, bath basin with warm water, bath thermometer, soap, 2-4 wash-cloths or disposable wipes, towel, gloves

1. Wash your hands.

2. Explain the procedure to the client, speaking clearly, slowly, and directly. Maintain face-to-face contact whenever possible.

3. Provide privacy for the client.

4. If the bed is adjustable, adjust bed to a safe level, usually waist high. If bed is movable, lock bed wheels.

5. Lower head of bed. Position client lying flat on her back.

6. Remove or fold back top bedding, keeping client covered with bath blanket.

7. Test water temperature with thermometer or on the inside of your wrist to ensure it is safe. Water temperature should be no higher than 105°F. Have client check water temperature. Adjust if necessary.

8. Put on gloves.

9. Ask the client to flex her knees and raise her buttocks off the bed by pushing against the mattress with her feet. Place clean protective pad under her buttocks.

10. Expose only the area necessary to clean the catheter. Avoid overexposing client.

11. Place towel or pad under catheter tubing before washing.

12. Wet washcloth in basin. Apply soap to washcloth. Clean area around meatus. Use a clean area of the washcloth for each stroke.

13. Hold catheter near meatus to avoid tugging the catheter.

14. Clean at least four inches of catheter nearest meatus. Move in only one direction, away from the meatus. Use a clean area of the cloth for each stroke.

15. Dip a clean washcloth in the water. Rinse area around meatus, using a clean area of washcloth for each stroke.

16. Dip a clean washcloth in the water. Rinse at least four inches of catheter nearest the meatus. Move in only one direction, away from the meatus (Fig. 4-88). Use a clean area of the cloth for each stroke.

17. With towel, dry at least four inches of catheter nearest meatus. Move in only one direction, away from meatus.

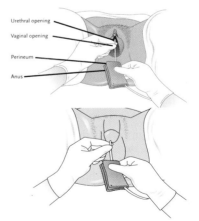

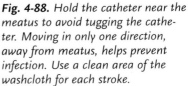

Fig. 4-88. Hold the catheter near the meatus to avoid tugging the catheter. Moving in only one direction, away from meatus, helps prevent infection. Use a clean area of the washcloth for each stroke.

18. Remove pad from under client. Remove towel or pad from under catheter tubing. Replace top covers and remove bath blanket.

19. Place soiled linen, towel, and washcloths in hamper. Empty basin into the toilet and flush. Clean, dry, and store the basin. Store supplies.

20. If you raised an adjustable bed, return it to its lowest position.

21. Remove and discard gloves.

22. Wash your hands.

23. Help the client dress. Arrange covers. Check that the catheter tubing is free from kinks and twists and that it is securely taped to the leg.

24. Wash your hands again.

25. Document procedure and any observations.

Emptying the catheter drainage bag

Equipment: graduate (measuring container), alcohol wipes, paper towels, gloves

1. Wash your hands.

2. Explain the procedure to the client, speaking clearly, slowly, and directly. Maintain face-to-face contact whenever possible.

3. Provide privacy for the client.

4. Put on gloves.

5. Place paper towel on the floor under the drainage bag. Place graduate on the paper towel.

6. Open the drain or spout on the bag so that urine flows out of the bag and into the graduate (Fig. 4-89). Do not let spout or clamp touch the graduate.

7. When urine has drained, close spout. Using alcohol wipe, clean the drain spout. Replace the drain in its holder on the bag.

8. Mentally note the amount and the appearance of the urine. Empty into toilet.

9. Go into the bathroom. Place graduate on a flat surface and measure at eye level. Note the amount and the appearance of the urine. Empty into toilet and flush toilet.

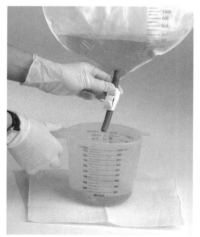

Fig. 4-89. Keep the spout from touching the graduate while draining urine.

10. Clean and store graduate. Discard paper towels.

11. Remove and discard gloves.

12. Wash your hands.

13. Document procedure. Note amount and characteristics of urine.

Ostomy Care

An **ostomy** is the surgical creation of an opening from an area inside the body to the outside. The terms *colostomy* and *ileostomy* refer to the surgical removal of a portion of the intestines. In a client with one of these ostomies, the end of the intestine is brought out of the body through an artificial opening in the abdomen. This opening is called a **stoma**. Stool, or feces, is eliminated through the ostomy rather than through the anus. An ostomy may be necessary due to bowel disease, cancer, or trauma.

The terms *colostomy* and *ileostomy* tell what part of the intestine was removed and the type of stool that will be eliminated. A **colostomy** is a surgically-created opening into the large intestine to allow stool to be expelled. With a colostomy, stool will generally be semi-solid. An ileostomy is a surgically-created opening into the end of the small intestine to allow stool to be expelled. Stool will be liquid and may be irritating to the client's skin.

Clients who have had an ostomy wear a disposable drainage bag that fits over the stoma to collect the feces. The bag is attached to the skin by adhesive. A belt may also be used to secure it.

Many people manage the ostomy appliance by themselves. If an HHA is providing ostomy care, she should give careful skin care. The ostomy bag should be emptied and cleaned or replaced whenever stool is eliminated. HHAs should always wear gloves and wash hands carefully when providing ostomy care. They can help by teaching proper handwashing to clients with ostomies.

Many clients with ostomies feel they have lost control of a basic bodily function. They may be embarrassed or angry about the ostomy. HHAs should be sensitive and supportive and should always provide privacy for ostomy care.

Providing ostomy care

Equipment: protective pad, bath blanket, clean ostomy drainage bag and belt, disposable wipes, basin of warm water, soap, washcloth, skin cream as ordered, 2 towels, plastic disposable bag, gloves

1. Wash your hands.

2. Explain the procedure to the client, speaking clearly, slowly, and directly. Maintain face-to-face contact whenever possible.

3. Provide privacy for the client.

4. If the bed is adjustable, adjust bed to a safe level, usually waist high. If bed is movable, lock bed wheels.

5. Put on gloves.

6. Place protective pad under client. Cover client with a bath blanket. Pull down the top sheet and blankets. Expose

only the ostomy site. Offer client a towel to keep clothing dry.

7. Remove ostomy bag carefully. Place it in the plastic bag. Note the color, odor, consistency, and amount of stool in the bag.

8. Wipe the area around the stoma with disposable wipes. Discard wipes in plastic bag.

9. Using a washcloth and warm, soapy water, wash the area in one direction, away from the stoma (Fig. 4-90). Rinse. Pat dry with another towel. Apply skin cream as ordered.

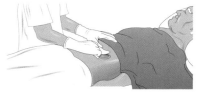

Fig. 4-90. *Wash area gently, moving away from the stoma.*

10. Place the clean ostomy appliance on client. Hold in place and seal securely. Make sure the bottom of the bag is clamped.

11. Remove protective pad and discard. Place soiled linens, washcloth, and towels in hamper. Discard plastic bag properly.

12. Remove and discard gloves.

13. Wash your hands.

14. Make the client comfortable and cover the client.

15. Return bed to lowest position if adjusted.

16. Document procedure and any observations. Note any changes in stoma and surrounding area. A normal stoma is red and moist and looks like the lining of the mouth. Call the supervisor if the stoma is very red or blue or if swelling or bleeding is present.

Collecting Specimens

HHAs may need to collect a specimen from a client. A **specimen** is a sample that is used for analysis in order to try to make a diagnosis. Different types of specimens that HHAs may be asked to collect include the following:

- Sputum (mucus coughed up from the lungs)
- Stool (feces)
- Urine (routine, clean-catch/mid-stream, or 24-hour)

Some clients will be able to collect their own specimens, while others will need help. The HHA should explain exactly how the specimen must be collected. All specimens must be labeled with the client's first and last name, date of birth, address, and the date and time the specimen was collected.

Sputum specimens may help diagnose respiratory problems or illness or evaluate the effects of medication. Early morning is the best time to collect sputum. The client should cough up the sputum and spit it directly into the specimen container. Proper personal protective equipment (PPE) must be worn when collecting sputum. The required PPE are gloves and a mask. The HHA's hands and the specimen container must be clean before beginning this procedure.

Collecting a sputum specimen

Equipment: specimen container with completed label (labeled with client's name, date of birth, address, date, and time) and lid, specimen bag or plastic bag, tissues, gloves, mask

1. Wash your hands.

2. Explain the procedure to the client, speaking clearly, slowly, and directly. Maintain face-to-face contact whenever possible.

3. Provide privacy for the client.

4. Put on mask and gloves. Coughing is one way that TB bacilli can enter the air. Stand behind the client if the client can hold the specimen container by himself.

5. Ask the client to cough deeply, so that sputum comes up from the lungs. To prevent the spread of infectious material, give the client tissues to cover his mouth while coughing. Ask the client to spit the sputum into the specimen container.

6. When you have obtained a good sample (about two table-spoons of sputum), cover the container tightly. Wipe any sputum off the outside of the container with tissues. Discard the tissues. Apply label, and place the specimen container in a clean specimen bag or plastic bag.

7. Remove and discard gloves and mask.

8. Wash your hands.

9. Document the procedure.

Stool (feces) specimens are collected so that the stool can be tested for blood, pathogens, and other things, such as worms or amoebas. The HHA should ask the client to let her know when he is ready to have a bowel movement, and she should be ready to collect the specimen.

Collecting a stool specimen

Equipment: specimen container with completed label (labeled with client's name, date of birth, address, date, and time) and lid, specimen bag, plastic bag, 2 tongue blades, 2 pairs of gloves, bedpan (if client cannot use a portable commode or toilet), hat for toilet (if client uses portable commode or toilet), toilet paper, disposable wipes, paper towels, supplies for perineal care

1. Wash your hands.

2. Explain the procedure to the client, speaking clearly, slowly, and directly. Maintain face-to-face contact whenever possible.

3. Provide privacy for the client.

4. Put on gloves.

5. Fit hat to toilet or commode, or provide client with bedpan.

6. Ask the client not to urinate when he is ready to move bowels. Ask him not to put toilet paper in with the sample. Provide a plastic bag to discard toilet paper separately.

7. Place toilet paper and disposable wipes within client's reach. Ask client to clean his hands with a wipe when finished if he is able.

8. Remove and discard gloves. Wash your hands.

9. Place a bell or other way to call you within client's reach. Ask the client to signal when done and explain that you will return when called. Leave the room and close the door.

10. When called by the client, return and put on clean gloves. Give perineal care if help is needed.

11. Using the two tongue blades, take about two tablespoons of stool and put it in the container. Without touching the inside of the container, cover it tightly.

Apply label, and place the specimen container in a clean specimen bag or plastic bag.

12. Wrap the tongue blades in toilet paper. Put them in plastic bag with used toilet paper. Discard bag in proper container.

13. Empty the bedpan or container into the toilet. Using a paper towel, turn on the faucet. Rinse the bedpan or container with cold water and empty it into the toilet. Flush the toilet. Then clean the bedpan or container with hot, soapy water and store.

14. Remove and discard gloves.

15. Wash your hands.

16. Document the procedure. Note amount and characteristics of stool.

Collecting a routine urine specimen

Equipment: specimen container with completed label (labeled with client's name, date of birth, address, date, and time) and lid, specimen bag, 2 pairs of gloves, bedpan or urinal (if client cannot use a portable commode or toilet), hat for toilet (if client uses portable commode or toilet), plastic bag, toilet paper, disposable wipes, paper towels, supplies for perineal care

1. Wash your hands.

2. Explain the procedure to the client, speaking clearly, slowly, and directly. Maintain face-to-face contact whenever possible.

3. Provide privacy for the client.

4. Put on gloves.

5. Fit hat to toilet or commode, or provide client with bedpan.

6. Ask client to void into hat, urinal, or bedpan. Ask the client not to put toilet paper in with the sample. Provide a plastic bag to discard toilet paper separately.

7. Place toilet paper and disposable wipes within client's reach. Ask client to clean his hands with a wipe when finished if he is able.

8. Remove and discard gloves. Wash your hands.

9. Place a bell or other way to call you within client's reach. Ask the client to signal when done and explain that you will return when called. Leave the room and close the door.

10. When called by the client, return and put on clean gloves.

Give perineal care if help is needed.

11. Take bedpan, urinal, or hat to the bathroom.

12. Pour urine into the specimen container. Specimen container should be at least half full.

13. Cover the urine container with its lid. Do not touch the inside of container. Wipe off the outside with a paper towel.

14. Apply label, and place the container in a clean specimen bag or plastic bag (Fig. 4-91).

15. Discard extra urine in the toilet. Using a paper towel, turn on the faucet. Rinse the bedpan, urinal, or hat with cold water and empty it into the toilet. Flush the toilet. Store the equipment.

16. Remove and discard gloves.

17. Wash your hands.

18. Document the procedure. Note amount and characteristics of urine.

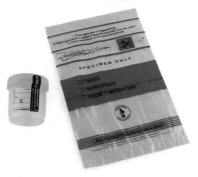

Fig. 4-91. *A specimen may need to be placed in a clean specimen bag or a plastic bag.*

Collecting a clean-catch (mid-stream) urine specimen

Equipment: specimen container with completed label (labeled with client's name, date of birth, address, date, and time) and lid, specimen bag, cleaning solution, gloves, bedpan or urinal (if client cannot use a portable commode or toilet), plastic bag, toilet paper, disposable wipes, paper towels, supplies for perineal care

1. Wash your hands.

2. Explain the procedure to the client, speaking clearly, slowly, and directly. Maintain face-to-face contact whenever possible.

3. Provide privacy for the client.

4. Put on gloves.

5. Open the specimen kit. Do not touch the inside of the container or the inside of the lid.

6. If client cannot clean his or her perineal area, you will need to do it. Use the wipes and cleaning solution to do this. Use a clean area of the wipe or clean wipe for each stroke. See bed bath procedure earlier in this chapter for reminder on how to give perineal care.

7. Ask the client to urinate a small amount into the bedpan, urinal, or toilet, and to stop before urination is complete.

8. Place the container under the urine stream and have the client start urinating again. Fill the container at least half full. Ask the client to stop urinating and remove the container. Have the client finish urinating in bedpan, urinal, or toilet.

9. After urination, provide a plastic bag so client can discard toilet paper. Give perineal care if help is needed. Ask client to

clean his hands with a wipe if he is able.

10. Cover the urine container with its lid. Do not touch the inside of the container. Wipe off the outside with a paper towel.

11. Apply label, and place the container in a clean specimen bag or plastic bag.

12. Discard extra urine in the toilet. Using a paper towel, turn on the faucet. Rinse the bedpan, urinal, or hat with cold water and empty it into the toilet. Flush the toilet. Store the equipment.

13. Remove and discard gloves.

14. Wash your hands.

15. Document the procedure. Note amount and characteristics of urine.

A 24-hour urine specimen collects all the urine voided by a client in a 24-hour period. The HHA will probably not be present during all 24 hours of the test, so it is important that he explain the collection fully to the client and family members.

Collecting a 24-hour urine specimen

Equipment: container for urine—gallon bottle or a container with lid from the lab, bedpan or urinal (if client cannot use a portable commode or toilet), hat for toilet (if client uses portable commode or toilet), bucket of ice (if the urine must be kept cold; a clearly-marked container can also be put in the refrigerator), funnel (if the container opening is small), gloves, disposable wipes, supplies for perineal care

1. Wash your hands.

2. Explain the procedure to the client, speaking clearly, slowly, and directly. Maintain face-to-face contact whenever possible.

3. Provide privacy for the client.

4. When starting the collection, have the client completely empty the bladder. Discard the urine and note the exact time of this voiding. The collection will run until the same time the next day.

5. Label the container with client's name, date of birth, address, and dates and times the collection period begins and ends.

6. Wash hands and put on gloves each time the client voids.

7. Pour urine from bedpan, urinal, or hat into the container, using the funnel as needed. Container may be stored at room temperature, in the refrigerator, or on ice. Follow the care plan's instructions.

8. After each voiding, assist as necessary with perineal care. Ask the client to clean his hands with a wipe after each voiding.

9. Be sure the client or a family member understands that all urine is to be saved, even when you are gone. Demonstrate how to pour the urine into the container. Remind them to store the container in the bucket of ice or in the refrigerator if ordered.

10. After each voiding, clean equipment.

11. Remove and discard gloves.

12. Wash your hands.

13. Document the time of the last void before the 24-hour collection period began, and the last void of the 24-hour collection period.

Non-Sterile Dressings

Sterile dressings cover open or draining wounds. A nurse changes these dressings. Non-sterile dressings are applied to dry, closed wounds that have less chance of infection. Home health aides may assist with non-sterile dressing changes.

Changing a dry dressing using non-sterile technique

Equipment: package of square gauze dressings, adhesive tape, scissors, 2 pairs of gloves, waste bag

1. Wash your hands.

2. Explain the procedure to the client, speaking clearly, slowly, and directly. Maintain face-to-face contact whenever possible.

3. Provide privacy for the client.

4. Cut pieces of tape long enough to secure the dressing. Hang tape on the edge of a table within reach. Open the four-inch square gauze package without touching the gauze. Place the opened package on a flat surface.

5. Put on gloves.

6. Remove soiled dressing by gently peeling tape toward the wound. Lift dressing off the wound. Do not drag it over the wound. Observe the dressing for any odor or drainage. Notice the color and size of the wound. Dispose of used dressing in the waste bag.

7. Remove and discard gloves. Place them in the waste bag. Wash your hands.

8. Put on new gloves. Touching only outer edges of new four-inch gauze, remove it from package. Apply it to the wound. Tape gauze in place. Secure it firmly (Fig. 4-92).

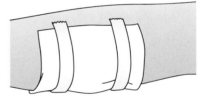

Fig. 4-92. Tape gauze in place to secure the dressing. Do not completely cover all areas of the dressing with tape.

9. Remove and discard gloves in the waste bag.

10. Wash your hands.

11. Document the procedure and your observations.

Warm and Cold Applications

Applying heat or cold to injured areas can have several positive effects. Heat relieves pain and muscular tension. It reduces swelling, elevates the temperature in the tissues, and increases blood flow. Increased blood flow brings more oxygen and nutrients to the tissues for healing. Cold applications can help stop bleeding. They help prevent swelling, reduce pain, and bring down high fevers. Applying ice bags or cold compresses immediately after an injury can stop bleeding and prevent swelling.

Warm and cold applications may be dry or moist. Moisture strengthens the effect of heat and cold. This means that moist applications are more likely to cause injury. Paralysis, numbness, disorientation, confusion, dementia, and other conditions may cause a person not to be able to feel, notice, or understand damage that is occurring from a warm or cold application. Home health aides must be careful when using these applications. They should know how long the application should be performed and should use the correct temperature as listed in the care plan. Clients receiving warm or cold applications should be checked often, as directed.

Observing and Reporting: Warm and Cold Applications

These signs indicate that the application may be causing tissue damage:

O/R Excessive redness

O/R Pain

O/R Blisters

O/R Numbness

Electric heating pads can be used as heat applications. An HHA should not use a heating pad unless it has been ordered in the care plan or by her supervisor.

Guidelines: Electric Heating Pad

G Check the skin frequently for redness or pain. Electric heating pads do not cool down. Having it just a little too hot can be very dangerous for the client.

G Make sure any electric heating pad you use is in good shape. Do not use it if the cord is frayed or if wires are exposed.

G Do not use a pin to fasten the pad. The pin could contact a wire inside the pad and cause a shock.

G Do not allow the client to lie on top of an electric heating pad.

G Do not allow the client to use an electric heating pad near a source of water.

A washcloth or a commercial warm compress may be used as a warm compress. If a commercial compress is provided, the HHA should follow the package directions and the supervisor's instructions.

Applying warm compresses

Equipment: washcloth or compress, plastic wrap, towel, basin, bath thermometer

1. Wash your hands.

2. Explain the procedure to the client, speaking clearly, slowly, and directly. Maintain face-to-face contact whenever possible.

3. Provide privacy for the client.

4. Fill basin one-half to two-thirds full with warm water. Test water temperature with thermometer or against the inside of your wrist to ensure it is safe. Water temperature should be no higher than 105°F. Have client check water temperature. Adjust if necessary.

5. Soak the washcloth in the water and wring it out. Immediately apply it to the area needing a warm compress. Note the time. Quickly cover the washcloth with plastic wrap and the towel to keep it warm (Fig. 4-93).

6. Check the area every five minutes. Remove the compress if the area is red or numb or if

the client complains of pain or discomfort. Change the compress if cooling occurs. Remove the compress after 20 minutes.

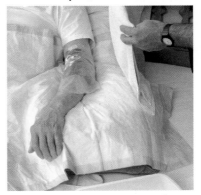

Fig. 4-93. Cover compresses to keep them warm.

7. Discard water in the toilet and flush the toilet. Rinse and wipe basin. Store basin and other supplies. Put soiled towels in hamper. Discard plastic wrap.

8. Wash your hands.

9. Document the time, length, and site of procedure, and any observations.

Administering warm soaks

Equipment: basin or bathtub (depending on the area to be soaked), bath thermometer, bath blanket, towel

1. Wash your hands.

2. Explain the procedure to the client, speaking clearly, slowly, and directly. Maintain face-to-face contact whenever possible.

3. Provide privacy for the client.

4. Fill the basin or tub half full of warm water. Test water temperature with thermometer or against the inside of your wrist to ensure it is safe. Water temperature should be no higher than 105°F. Have client check water temperature. Adjust if necessary.

5. Immerse the body part in the basin, or help the client into the tub. Pad the edge of the basin with a towel (Fig. 4-94). Use a bath blanket to cover the client if needed for extra warmth.

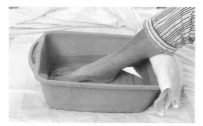

Fig. 4-94. *Pad the edge of the basin to make the client more comfortable.*

6. Check water temperature every five minutes. Add hot water as needed to maintain the temperature. Never add water hotter than 105°F to avoid burns. To prevent burns, ask the client not to add hot water. Observe the area for redness. Discontinue the soak if the client complains of pain or discomfort.

7. Soak for 15 to 20 minutes or as ordered.

8. Remove basin or help the client out of the tub. Use the towel to dry client.

9. Drain the tub or discard water. Rinse and wipe basin. Store basin and other supplies. Put soiled towel in hamper.

10. Wash your hands.

11. Document the time, length, and site of procedure. Report the client's response and any of your observations about the skin.

Another type of heat application is a sitz bath, or a warm soak of the perineal area. Sitz baths clean perineal wounds and reduce inflammation and pain. Circulation in the perineal area is increased. Voiding may be stimulated by a sitz bath. Clients with perineal swelling (such as hemorrhoids), or perineal wounds (such as those that occur during childbirth), may be ordered to take sitz baths. A disposable sitz bath fits on the toilet seat and is attached to a rubber bag containing warm water (Fig. 4-95). Because the sitz bath causes increased blood flow to the pelvic area, blood flow to other parts of the body is decreased. Clients may feel weak, faint, or dizzy after a sitz bath. HHAs must always wear gloves when helping with a sitz bath.

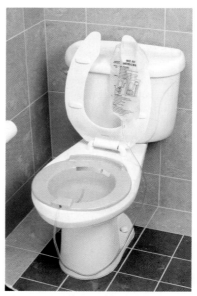

Fig. 4-95. *A disposable sitz bath.*
(REPRINTED WITH PERMISSION OF BRIGGS CORPORATION, 800-247-2343, WWW.BRIGGSCORP.COM)

Assisting with a sitz bath

Equipment: disposable sitz bath, bath thermometer, towels, gloves

1. Wash your hands.

2. Explain the procedure to the client, speaking clearly, slowly, and directly. Maintain face-to-face contact whenever possible.

3. Provide privacy for the client.

4. Put on gloves.

5. Fill the sitz bath two-thirds full with warm water. Place the disposable sitz bath on the toilet seat. Check the water temperature using the bath thermometer. Water temperature should be no higher than 105°F. If the sitz bath is being used to help relieve pain and to stimulate circulation, the water temperature may need to be higher. Follow instructions in the care plan.

6. Help the client undress and sit on the sitz bath. A valve on the tubing connected to the bag allows the client or you to refill the water in the sitz bath again with warm water.

7. You may be required to stay with the client for safety reasons. If you leave the room, check on the client every five minutes to make sure he or she is not dizzy or weak. Stay with a client who seems unsteady.

8. Help the client off of the sitz bath after 20 minutes. Provide towels and help with dressing if needed.

9. Place soiled towel in hamper. Clean and store supplies.

10. Remove and discard gloves.

11. Wash your hands.

12. Document the procedure, including the time started and ended, the client's response, and the water temperature.

Applying ice packs

Equipment: cold pack or sealable plastic bag and crushed ice, towel to cover pack or bag

1. Wash your hands.

2. Explain the procedure to the client, speaking clearly, slowly, and directly. Maintain face-to-face contact whenever possible.

3. Provide privacy for the client.

4. Fill plastic bag one-half to two-thirds full with crushed ice. Seal bag. Remove excess air. Cover bag with towel (Fig. 4-96).

5. Apply bag to the area. Note the time. Use another towel to cover bag if it is too cold.

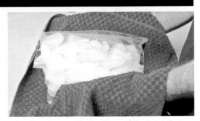

Fig. 4-96. *Seal the bag filled with ice and cover it with a towel.*

6. Check the area after 10 minutes for blisters, pale, white, or gray skin. Stop treatment if client complains of numbness or pain.

7. Remove ice after 20 minutes or as ordered in the care plan.

8. Place soiled towel in hamper. Discard supplies or store in freezer if ordered.

9. Wash your hands.

10. Document the time, length, and site of procedure. Report the client's response and any of your observations about the skin.

Applying cold compresses

Equipment: basin filled with water and ice, 2 washcloths, protective pad, towels

1. Wash your hands.

2. Explain the procedure to the client, speaking clearly, slowly, and directly. Maintain face-to-face contact whenever possible.

3. Provide privacy for the client.

4. Place protective pad under area to be treated. Rinse washcloth in basin and wring out (Fig. 4-97). Cover the area to be treated with a towel. Apply cold washcloth to the area as directed. Change washcloths often to keep area cold.

5. Check the area after five minutes for blisters or pale, white, or gray skin. Stop treatment if client complains of numbness or pain.

6. Remove compresses after 20 minutes or as ordered in the care plan. Give client towels as needed to dry the area.

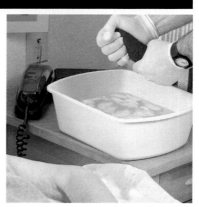

Fig. 4-97. Wring out the washcloth before applying it to the area to be treated.

7. Place soiled towels in hamper. Discard protective pad. Discard water, and rinse and wipe basin. Store basin.

8. Wash your hands.

9. Document the time, length, and site of procedure. Report the client's response and any observations about the skin.

Medications

People who need home care often need medications. HHAs do not usually handle or give medications. However, HHAs need to understand the kinds of medicine that clients may be taking. It is also important to know what to do if a client experiences side effects or refuses to take medication. If a client is taking medications that can be purchased over-the-counter (OTC) or without a physician's prescription, the HHA should notify the supervisor. Sometimes OTC medications interfere with the desired effects of prescription medications.

Many states have passed laws regarding the responsibilities and limitations for helping clients with medications. HHAs must know the regulations in their state and only provide assistance that is allowed.

Guidelines: Safe and Proper Use of Medications

G   Never handle or give medications unless you are specifically trained and assigned to do so. Do not touch the inside of a medicine bottle or the pills or other medicines themselves. Do not put any medication in a client's mouth. Handling or giving medication can have serious consequences.

G   Observe clients taking their medication. Although you cannot handle or give medication, you can remind clients to take their medications. You can also bring medication containers to clients, and provide water or food as needed to take with the medication. Always observe, report, and document as appropriate.

G   Know the difference between prescription drugs and non-prescription (over-the-counter) drugs. Antibiotics (such as penicillin), heart drugs (such as nitroglycerin), and potent pain medication (such as codeine) are examples of prescription drugs. Aspirin and cold medications, such as decongestants, are over-the-counter drugs.

G   Be aware of all medications a client is taking. There are many possible side effects and interactions among medications. Watch for symptoms such as itching, trembling or shaking, anxiety, stomachache, diarrhea, confusion, vomiting, rash, hives, or headache. Any of these symptoms could indicate a side effect or interaction. Report any of these symptoms to your supervisor.

Knowing and remembering the five "rights" of medications will help prevent mistakes.

1. The Right Client

2. The Right Medication

3. The Right Time

4. The Right Route (how the medication should be taken)

5. The Right Amount

An HHA should call her supervisor if the medication label and the care plan do not agree on any of the five "rights." She should also call her supervisor if there is not enough information on the label or in the care plan, or if there is another problem with the medication (for example, the client's name is not on the container).

If a client shows signs of a reaction to a medication, or complains of side effects, the HHA must report it right away. The supervisor can assess whether or not the symptom is caused by the medication. The HHA's responsibility is to report her observations.

Observing and Reporting: Medications

O/R Dizziness, fainting

O/R Nausea, vomiting, diarrhea

O/R Rash, hives, itching

O/R Difficulty breathing, swelling of throat or eyes

O/R Drowsiness

O/R Headache, blurred vision

O/R Abdominal pain

O/R Any other unusual sign

In addition, report any of the following problems immediately:

O/R Client refuses to take medication as directed.

O/R Client takes the wrong dose (amount) of medication.

O/R Client takes medication at the wrong time.

O/R Client takes the wrong medication.

O/R A medication container is missing or empty.

If a client has difficulty swallowing the medication, the HHA should report it to the supervisor. The doctor can then make appropriate changes. The HHA should never crush tablets or empty capsules of medications into the client's food or drink.

If a client has a severe allergic reaction to a medication, takes the wrong dose, or takes medications together that cause complications, emergency medical treatment is necessary. An overdose, whether it was accidental or intentional, must be treated as a poisoning. The HHA must call the Poison Control Center number immediately and follow their instructions. Poison Control will send paramedics if needed. For severe drug reactions or interactions, the HHA should call 911 or 0 for emergency help. She should stay with the client and not give any liquids, food, or other medications unless instructed to do so by emergency personnel. The supervisor should be notified as soon as possible.

When assisting with the proper storage of medications, the HHA should follow these guidelines:

Guidelines: Proper Storage of Medications

G Keep the client's medications in one place, separate from medicine used by other members of the household.

G If there are young children or a disoriented elderly person in the home, medications should be locked away.

G All medications should be kept in childproof containers if children are in the home. To avoid an accidental overdose, keep medications out of reach of children.

G If medicine requires refrigeration, store the bottle on an upper shelf toward the back, out of a child's reach.

G Store all medications away from heat and light.

G The client or family member should discard medications that have expired, are not labeled, or are discolored. Make sure these medications are not discarded in the trash. Children or animals may have access to them. Ask your supervisor for specific disposal instructions if the client or family will not dispose of expired medications. Do not dispose of them yourself.

Drug misuse and abuse may be accidental or deliberate. It includes the following:

- Refusing to take medications
- Taking the wrong dose or taking it at the wrong time
- Mixing medication with alcohol
- Taking drugs that have not been prescribed
- Taking illegal drugs
- Sharing drugs with others

Misuse or abuse of drugs is extremely dangerous and can even be fatal. HHAs should be alert to the signs of misuse or abuse and report them to their supervisor immediately.

Observing and Reporting: Drug Misuse and Abuse

O/R Depression

O/R Anorexia

O/R Change in sleep patterns

O/R Withdrawn behavior or moodiness

O/R Secrecy

O/R   Verbal abusiveness

O/R   Poor relationships with family members

The drugs that pose the highest risk for causing drug dependency are pain medications, tranquilizers, muscle relaxers, and sleeping pills. Substance abuse is the use of legal or illegal drugs, cigarettes, or alcohol in a way that harms oneself or others. It is not necessary for a substance to be illegal for it to be abused. Alcohol and cigarettes are legal for adults, but are often abused. Over-the-counter medications, including diet aids and decongestants, can be addictive and harmful. Even household substances such as paint or glue are sometimes abused, causing injury and death.

HHAs may be in a position to observe signs of substance abuse in clients. These signs should be reported to the supervisor. HHAs can report their observations without accusing anyone. They should simply report what they see, not what they think the cause may be.

Observing and Reporting: Substance Abuse

O/R   Changes in physical appearance (red eyes, dilated pupils, weight loss)

O/R   Changes in personality (moodiness, strange behavior, disruption of routines, lying)

O/R   Irritability

O/R   Odor of cigarettes, liquor, or other substances on breath or clothes

O/R   Diminished sense of smell

O/R   Unexplained changes in vital signs

O/R   Loss of appetite

O/R   Inability to function normally

O/R   Confusion or forgetfulness

O/R   Blackouts or memory loss

O/R   Frequent accidents

O/R   Need for money, or money missing from the home

O/R   Alcohol or cigarettes missing from the home

O/R   Problems with family or friends

O/R   New friends or companions, strange phone calls

Oxygen

Clients may receive oxygen therapy. **Oxygen therapy** is the administration of oxygen to increase the supply of oxygen to the lungs. This increases oxygen to the body tissues. Oxygen therapy is used to treat breathing difficulties and is prescribed by a doctor. Home health aides never stop, adjust, or administer oxygen.

Oxygen will be delivered to the home in tanks or produced by an oxygen concentrator. Compressed oxygen and liquid oxygen are stored in tanks of varying sizes. An oxygen concentrator produces and distributes oxygen, but does not store oxygen. The agency that supplies the oxygen will service the equipment and will provide training on its use.

An oxygen concentrator is a box-like device that changes air in the room into air with more oxygen. Oxygen concentrators are quiet machines. They can be larger units or portable ones that can move or travel with the client. Oxygen concentrators run on electricity. They are plugged into wall outlets and are turned on and off by a switch. It may take several minutes for the oxygen concentrator to reach full power after it is turned on.

Some clients receive oxygen through a nasal cannula. A nasal cannula is a piece of plastic tubing that fits around the face and is secured by a strap that goes over the ears and around the back of the head. The face piece has two short, curved prongs made of tubing. These prongs fit inside the nose, and oxygen is delivered through them. A nurse or respiratory therapist fits the cannula. The length of the prongs (usually no more than half an inch) is adjusted for the client's comfort. The client can talk and eat while wearing the cannula (Fig. 4-98).

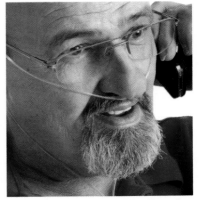

Fig. 4-98. Clients can still talk and eat while wearing a nasal cannula.

Clients who do not need concentrated oxygen all the time may use a face mask when they need oxygen. The face mask fits over the nose and mouth. It is secured by a strap that goes over the ears and around the back of the head. The mask should be checked to see that it fits snugly on the client's face, but it should not pinch the face. It is difficult for a client to talk while wearing an oxygen face mask. The mask must be removed for the client to eat or drink anything.

Oxygen can be irritating to the nose and mouth. The strap of a nasal cannula or face mask can also cause irritation around the ears. HHAs should wash and dry skin carefully and provide frequent mouth care. They should offer clients plenty of fluids and report any irritation observed.

Combustion means the process of burning. Oxygen is a very dangerous fire hazard because it supports combustion (makes other things burn). Working around oxygen requires special safety precautions.

Guidelines: Working Safely Around Oxygen

G   Post *No Smoking* and *Oxygen in Use* signs. Never allow smoking in the room or area where oxygen is used or stored.

G   Remove all fire hazards from the area. Fire hazards include electrical equipment, such as electrical razors and hair dryers. Cigarettes, matches, and flammable fluids are also fire hazards. **Flammable** means easily ignited and capable of burning quickly. Alcohol and nail polish remover are examples of flammable liquids. Notify your supervisor if a client does not want a fire hazard removed.

G   Do not burn candles, light matches, or use lighters around oxygen.

G   Do not use an extension cord with an oxygen concentrator.

G   Do not place electrical cords or oxygen tubing under rugs or furniture.

G   Avoid using fabrics such as nylon and wool that can cause static electricity discharges.

G   Report if the nasal cannula or face mask causes skin irritation. Check the nasal area and behind the ears for signs of irritation.

G   Do not use any petroleum-based products, such as Vaseline or Chapstick, on the client or on any part of the cannula or mask.

G   Learn how to turn off oxygen in case of fire. Never adjust the oxygen setting or dose.

IVs

Intravenous therapy, often called *IV therapy*, is the delivery of medication, nutrition, or fluids through a person's vein. IV is the abbreviation for **intravenous**, or into a vein. When a physician prescribes IV therapy, a nurse inserts a needle or tube into a vein. This allows direct access to the bloodstream. Medication, nutrition, or fluids either drip from a bag suspended on a pole or are pumped by a portable pump through a tube and into the vein. Some clients with chronic conditions may have a permanent opening for IV lines, called a *port*. This opening has been surgically created to allow easy access for IV fluids. HHAs never insert or remove IV lines. They are not responsible for care of the IV site. Their only responsibility for IV care is to report and document any observations of changes or problems with the IV.

Observing and Reporting: IVs

Report any of the following to your supervisor:

- ^O/R The tube/needle falls out or is removed
- ^O/R The tubing disconnects
- ^O/R The dressing around the IV site is loose or not intact
- ^O/R Blood is in the tubing or around the IV site
- ^O/R The site is swollen or discolored
- ^O/R The client complains of pain
- ^O/R The bag is broken, or the level of fluid does not seem to decrease
- ^O/R The IV fluid is not dripping or is leaking
- ^O/R The IV fluid is nearly gone
- ^O/R The pump beeps, indicating a problem
- ^O/R The pump is dropped

HHAs should not do any of the following when caring for a client who has an IV line:

- Measure blood pressure on an arm with an IV line
- Get the IV site wet
- Pull or catch the tubing in anything, such as clothing
- Leave the tubing kinked
- Lower the IV bag below the IV site
- Touch the clamp
- Disconnect the IV from the pump

V. Special Clients, Special Needs

Disabilities and Mental Illnesses

Disabilities

A disability is the impairment of a physical or mental function. Disability may result from a disease, a complication of pregnancy, or an injury. A disability can be temporary or it can be permanent. Depending on the disability, a person may not be able to perform activities of daily living (ADLs). Work and social activities may be limited. People with disabilities may be more susceptible to illness. By strictly following the care plan and carefully observing and reporting, HHAs can help clients with disabilities avoid illness and may also help clients lead more independent lives.

Families of people with disabilities may find it difficult to cope with the stress a disability can cause. They may feel resentment, disappointment, guilt, shame, anger, or frustration. Caring for someone with a disability can be a big responsibility. It affects a family's time, energy, patience, and financial resources. Home health aides can give family members a much-needed break. Clients and their families may need additional support, including counseling, to help deal with the disability. An HHA should report to his supervisor if he thinks additional support is needed.

Illness or disability requires clients and families to make adjustments. Making these adjustments may be difficult. It depends on the family's emotional, spiritual, and financial resources. Some personal adjustments include the following:

- Accepting the illness or disability and its long-term consequences or results
- Finding money to pay expenses of hospitalization or home care
- Dealing with paperwork required for insurance, Medicaid, or Medicare
- Taking care of tasks the client can no longer handle
- Understanding medical information and making difficult care decisions
- Providing daily care when the aide cannot be there
- Caring for children while caring for an elderly loved one (called the *sandwich generation*—being "sandwiched" between two generations)

G   Promote self-care and independence. Help your clients with disabilities do all they can for themselves. Give them opportunities to show what they can do. Do not take over a task just because you can do it faster or better. Feelings of independence, dignity, acceptance, social interaction, and self-worth are all boosted when the client is able to perform a task for himself. However, do not push a client beyond his or her abilities.

G   Assure the client's safety. Be aware of accidents that commonly occur in the home. Most can be avoided if you think ahead. Think critically about each client's abilities and disabilities. Safety concerns vary depending on the disability.

G   Promote the client's health and comfort. Help your clients by maintaining nutrition and hydration and by assisting with personal care. The care plan and your assignment sheet will include instructions for this type of care. To provide further comfort, watch and listen to the client.

G   Maintain the client's dignity and self-worth. Never discuss a client with anyone other than a member of the care team. Treat a client who is disabled with the same respect you would give any client. Be sensitive to the client's feelings. Find ways to make your clients feel good about themselves. Allow and encourage the client to direct how and when care is provided.

G   Maintain the stability of the client's household. Help maintain the stability of the household by being punctual and dependable. Respect the schedules of the family. Work cheerfully, calmly, and efficiently.

G   Observe, report, and document carefully. For clients with disabilities that affect mobility, be very careful to observe and report changes in the skin. Pressure ulcer prevention is an important role of the home health aide. Emotional changes should also be observed and reported. Clients may be at risk for depression. Report any signs of depression, including moodiness, weight loss or gain, fatigue, or withdrawal.

Mental Illnesses

Mental health is the normal functioning of emotional and intellectual abilities. A person who is mentally healthy is able to do the following:

- Get along with others
- Adapt to change

- Care for self and others
- Give and accept love
- Deal with situations that cause anxiety, disappointment, and frustration
- Take responsibility for decisions, feelings, and actions
- Control and fulfill desires and impulses appropriately

While it involves emotional and mental functioning, mental illness is a disorder. It produces signs and symptoms and affects the body's ability to function. It responds to proper treatment and care. Mental illness disrupts a person's ability to function at a normal level in the family, home, and community. It often causes inappropriate behavior. Some signs and symptoms of mental illness are confusion, disorientation, **agitation**, and anxiety. Mental illness can be caused or made worse by chronic stress from any of these conditions:

- Physical factors, such as illness, disability, aging, substance abuse, or chemical imbalance
- Environmental factors, such as weak interpersonal or family relationships or traumatic early life experiences
- Heredity
- Stress

A fallacy is a false belief. The greatest fallacy about mental illness is that people who are mentally ill can control it. Mentally ill people cannot simply choose to be well. People who are mentally healthy are usually able to control their emotions and actions. People who are mentally ill may not have this control.

Mental health is important to physical health. Reducing stress can help prevent some physical illnesses. It can help people cope if illness or disability occur. Mental health can help protect and improve physical health. The reverse is also true. Physical illness or disability can cause or worsen mental illness. The stress these conditions create takes a toll on mental health.

Different types of mental illness will affect how well clients communicate. HHAs should treat each client as an individual and tailor their approach to the situation.

Guidelines: Communication and Mental Illness

G Do not talk to adults as if they were children.

G Use simple, clear statements and a normal tone of voice.

G   Be sure that what you say and how you say it show respect and concern.

G   Sit or stand at a normal distance from the client. Be aware of your body language.

G   Be honest and direct, as you would with any client.

G   Avoid arguments.

G   Maintain eye contact and listen carefully.

There are many types of mental illness, ranging from mild to severe.

Anxiety Disorders: **Anxiety** is uneasiness or fear, often about a situation or condition. When a person who is mentally healthy feels anxiety, he usually knows the cause. The anxiety fades once the cause is removed. A person who is mentally ill may feel anxiety all the time. He may not know the reason why. Physical symptoms of anxiety disorders include shakiness, muscle aches, sweating, cold and clammy hands, dizziness, fatigue, racing heart, cold or hot flashes, a choking or smothering sensation, and a dry mouth.

Types of anxiety disorders include panic disorder, obsessive-compulsive disorder (OCD), post-traumatic stress disorder (PTSD), and phobias. With panic disorder, a person has repeated episodes of intense fear that something bad will occur. Obsessive-compulsive disorder is an anxiety disorder characterized by obsessive behavior or thoughts. For example, a person may wash his hands over and over as a way of dealing with anxiety. Post-traumatic stress disorder is an anxiety disorder caused by a traumatic experience. A **phobia** is an intense form of anxiety or fear. Many people are very afraid of certain things (for example, dogs or snakes) or situations (like being in a confined space, or flying). For a person with a mental illness, a phobia is a disabling terror. It prevents the person from participating in normal activities.

Mood Disorders: Many people feel sad, stressed, or irritable at times. However, a mood disorder affects a person's emotions on a daily basis. **Major depressive disorder**, also called *clinical depression* or *major depression*, is one type of mood disorder. It may cause intense mental, emotional, and physical pain and disability. This disorder also makes other illnesses worse. If untreated, it may result in suicide. Clinical depression is not a normal reaction to stress. Sadness is only one symptom of this illness. Not all people who have this disorder complain of sadness or appear sad. Other common symptoms of clinical depression include the following:

• Pain, including headaches, abdominal pain, and other body aches

• Low energy or fatigue

- Apathy, or lack of interest in activities
- Irritability
- Anxiety
- Loss of appetite or overeating
- Problems with sexual functioning and desire
- Sleeplessness, difficulty sleeping, or excessive sleeping
- Lack of attention to basic personal care tasks (e.g., bathing, combing hair, changing clothes)
- Intense feelings of despair
- Guilt
- Difficulty concentrating
- Withdrawal and isolation
- Repeated thoughts of suicide and death

Bipolar disorder, also called *manic-depressive illness*, is another type of mood disorder. Bipolar disorder causes a person to swing from deep depression to extreme activity. These episodes can include high energy, little sleep, big speeches, rapidly changing thoughts and moods, high self-esteem, overspending, and poor judgment.

Psychotic Disorders: Psychotic disorders are severe mental disorders that cause problems with perception and the ability to understand reality. **Schizophrenia** is a type of psychotic disorder that affects a person's ability to think and communicate clearly. It also affects the ability to manage emotions, make decisions, and understand reality. It affects a person's ability to interact with other people. Symptoms of schizophrenia include the following:

- Hallucinations
- Delusions
- Disorganized thinking and speech
- Moving slowly, repeating rhythmic gestures or movements
- Showing little emotion or interest
- Lack of energy

Guidelines: Mental Illness

G   Observe clients carefully for changes in condition or abilities. Document and report your observations.

G   Support the client and his family and friends. Your positive, professional attitude encourages them.

G   Encourage clients to do as much for themselves as possible. Progress may be very slow. Be patient, supportive, and positive.

G   Mental illness can be treated. Medication and psychotherapy are common methods of treatment. Medication must be taken properly to promote benefits and reduce side effects. Home health aides may be assigned to observe clients taking their medications. Psychotherapy is a method of treating mental illness that involves talking about one's problems with mental health professionals.

Observing and Reporting: Mental Illness

O/R   Changes in ability

O/R   Positive or negative mood changes, especially withdrawal

O/R   Behavior changes, including changes in personality, extreme behavior, and behavior that does not seem to fit the situation

O/R   Comments, even jokes, about hurting self or others

O/R   Failure to take medication or improper use of medication

O/R   Real or imagined physical symptoms

O/R   Events, situations, or people that seem to upset or excite clients

Special Conditions

Certain special conditions or diseases require specific types of care. A quick overview of these conditions follows:

- Arthritis
- Cancer
- Diabetes
- CVA or Stroke
- Multiple Sclerosis (MS)
- Circulatory Disorders
- HIV and AIDS
- Dementia
- Alzheimer's Disease (AD)
- Chronic Obstructive Pulmonary Disease (COPD)
- Tuberculosis (TB)
- Hip or Knee Replacement

Arthritis

Arthritis is a general term that refers to inflammation, or swelling, of the joints. It causes stiffness, pain, and decreased mobility. Arthritis may be the result of aging, injury, or an autoimmune illness. Autoimmune illnesses cause the body's immune system to attack normal tissue in the body. Two common types of arthritis are rheumatoid arthritis and osteoarthritis.

Rheumatoid arthritis can affect people of all ages. Joints become red, swollen, and very painful. Deformities can result and may be severe and disabling. Movement is eventually restricted. Fever, fatigue, and weight loss are also symptoms. Osteoarthritis, also called degenerative joint disease (DJD) or degenerative arthritis, often affects older people. It may occur with aging or as the result of joint injury. Hips and knees, which are weight-bearing joints, are usually affected. Joints in the fingers, thumbs, and spine can also be affected. Pain and stiffness seem to increase in cold or damp weather.

Arthritis is often treated with some or all of the following:

- Anti-inflammatory medications such as aspirin or ibuprofen, or other medication
- Local applications of heat to reduce swelling and pain
- Range of motion exercises
- Regular exercise and/or activity routines
- Diet to reduce weight or maintain strength

Guidelines: Arthritis

G   Watch for stomach irritation or heartburn caused by aspirin or ibuprofen. Some clients cannot take these medications. Report signs of stomach irritation or heartburn immediately.

G   Encourage activity. Gentle activity can help reduce the effects of arthritis. Follow the care plan instructions carefully. Use canes or other walking aids as needed.

G   Adapt activities of daily living (ADLs) to allow independence. Many devices are available to help clients bathe, dress, and feed themselves when they have arthritis.

G   Choose clothing that is easy to put on and fasten. Encourage use of handrails and safety bars in the bathroom.

G   Treat each client as an individual. Arthritis is very common among older clients. Do not assume that all clients have the same symptoms and need the same care.

G   Help maintain client's self-esteem by encouraging self-care. Have a positive attitude. Listen to the client's feelings. You can help him remain independent as long as possible.

Cancer

Cancer is a general term used to describe a disease in which abnormal cells grow in an uncontrolled way. Cancer usually occurs in the form of a tumor or tumors growing on or within the body. A **tumor** is a group of abnormally-growing cells. Benign tumors are considered non-cancerous. They usually grow slowly in local areas. Malignant tumors are cancerous. They can grow rapidly and invade surrounding tissues.

Cancer invades local tissue and can spread to other parts of the body. When cancer spreads from the site where it first appeared (metastasizes), it can affect other body systems. In general, treatment is more difficult and cancer is more deadly after this has occurred. Cancer often appears first in the breast, colon, rectum, uterus, prostate, lungs, or skin. There is no known cure for cancer, but some treatments are effective.

These risk factors may contribute to cancer:

- Age
- Race
- Gender
- Family history
- Tobacco use
- Alcohol use
- Poor diet/obesity
- Lack of physical activity
- Chemicals and food additives
- Radiation
- Exposure to sunlight

When diagnosed early, cancer can often be treated and controlled. The American Cancer Society (cancer.org) has identified some warning signs of cancer:

- Unexplained weight loss
- Fever

- Fatigue
- Pain
- Skin changes
- Change in bowel or bladder function
- Sores that do not heal
- Unusual bleeding or discharge
- Thickening or lump in the breast, scrotum, or other part of the body
- Indigestion or difficulty swallowing
- New mole or recent change in appearance of a mole or wart
- Nagging cough or hoarseness

People with cancer can often live longer and sometimes recover if they are treated early. Often these treatments are combined:

- Surgery
- Chemotherapy
- Radiation

Guidelines: Cancer

G   Each case is different. Cancer is a general term and refers to many separate situations. Clients may live many years or only several months. Treatment affects each person differently. Do not make assumptions about a client's condition.

G   Clients may want to talk or may avoid talking. Respect each client's needs. Be honest. Never say, "Everything will be okay." Be sensitive. Remember that cancer is a disease, and its cause is unknown.

G   Proper nutrition is very important for clients with cancer. Follow the care plan carefully. Clients frequently have poor appetites. Encourage a variety of food and small portions. Liquid nutrition supplements may be used in addition to, not in place of, meals. If nausea or swallowing is a problem, foods such as soups, gelatin, or starches may appeal to the client. Use plastic utensils for a client receiving chemotherapy. It makes food taste better. Metal utensils cause a bitter taste.

G   Cancer can cause great pain, especially in the late stages. Watch for signs of pain. Assist with comfort measures, such as back rubs, repositioning, and providing conversation, music, or reading materials. Report if pain seems to be uncontrolled.

G Give back rubs for comfort and to increase circulation. For clients who spend many hours in bed, moving to a chair for a period of time may improve comfort as well. Reposition weak or immobile clients at least every two hours.

G Use lotion regularly on dry or delicate skin. Do not apply lotion to areas receiving radiation therapy. Do not remove markings that are used in radiation therapy. Follow any skin care orders.

G Help clients brush and floss teeth regularly. Medications, nausea, vomiting, or mouth infections may cause pain and a bad taste in the mouth. You can help by using a soft-bristled toothbrush, rinsing with baking soda and water, or using a prescribed rinse. Do not use a commercial mouthwash. For clients with mouth sores, use oral swabs, rather than toothbrushes. Be gentle when giving care.

G People with cancer may have a poor self-image because they are weak and their appearance has changed. For example, hair loss is a common side effect of chemotherapy. Help with grooming if desired.

G If visitors help cheer your client, encourage them and do not intrude. If some times of day are better than others, suggest this to visitors.

G Caring for a person with cancer at home can be very difficult for family members. Be alert to needs that are not being met or stresses created by the illness. Report your observations.

G Report any of the following to your supervisor:

- Increased weakness or fatigue
- Weight loss
- Nausea, vomiting, or diarrhea
- Changes in appetite
- Fainting
- Signs of depression
- Confusion
- Blood in stool or urine
- Changes in mental status
- Changes in skin
- New lumps, sores, or rashes
- Increase in pain, or unrelieved pain
- Blood in the mouth

Numerous services and support groups are available for people with cancer and their families or caregivers. The *Important Names/Numbers* section, located at the end of this book, after the index, contains a list of community resources and their contact information.

Diabetes

Diabetes mellitus, commonly called **diabetes**, occurs when the pancreas produces too little insulin or does not properly use insulin. Insulin is a hormone that converts glucose, or natural sugar, into energy for the body. Without insulin to process glucose, these sugars collect in the blood and cannot get to cells. This causes problems with circulation and can damage vital organs.

Diabetes is common in people with a family history of the illness, in the elderly, and in people who are obese. Diabetes is a chronic disease that has two major types: type 1 and type 2.

Type 1 diabetes is usually diagnosed in children and young adults. In type 1 diabetes, the body does not produce any insulin. The condition will continue throughout a person's life. Type 1 diabetes is managed with daily injections of insulin or an insulin pump and a special diet. Regular blood glucose testing must be done.

Type 2 diabetes is the most common form of diabetes. In type 2 diabetes, either the body does not produce enough insulin or the body fails to properly use insulin. This is known as *insulin resistance*. Type 2 diabetes usually develops slowly. It is the milder form of diabetes. It typically develops after age 35. The risk of getting it increases with age. However, the number of children with type 2 diabetes is growing rapidly. Type 2 diabetes often occurs in obese people or those with a family history of the disease. It can usually be controlled with diet and/or oral medications. Blood glucose levels should be tested regularly.

Pre-diabetes occurs when a person's blood glucose levels are above normal but not high enough for a diagnosis of type 2 diabetes. Research indicates that some damage to the body, especially to the heart and circulatory system, may already be occurring during pre-diabetes. Pregnant women who have never had diabetes before but who have high blood sugar (glucose) levels during pregnancy are said to have *gestational diabetes*.

People with diabetes may have these signs and symptoms:

- Excessive thirst
- Extreme hunger
- Frequent urination
- Weight loss

- High blood sugar levels (hyperglycemia)
- Glucose (sugar) in the urine (glucosuria)
- Sudden vision changes
- Tingling or numbness in hands or feet (neuropathy)
- Feeling very tired much of the time
- Very dry skin
- Sores that are slow to heal
- More infections than usual

Diabetes can lead to further complications:

- Changes in the circulatory system can cause heart attack and stroke, reduced circulation, poor wound healing, and kidney and nerve damage.
- Damage to the eyes can cause vision loss and blindness.
- Poor circulation and impaired wound healing may cause leg and foot ulcers, infected wounds, and gangrene. Gangrene can lead to amputation.
- Insulin reaction and diabetic ketoacidosis can be serious complications of diabetes. *Medical Emergencies* in Section II contains more information about these conditions.

Diabetes must be carefully controlled to prevent complications and severe illness. When working with clients with diabetes, HHAs must follow care plan instructions carefully.

Guidelines: Caring for Clients with Diabetes

G   Follow diet instructions exactly. The intake of carbohydrates, including breads, potatoes, grains, pasta, and sugars, must be regulated. Meals must be eaten at the same time each day. The client must eat all that is served. If a client will not eat what is served, or if you suspect that he is not following the diet when you leave, report this to your supervisor.

G   Encourage the client to follow his exercise program. Regular exercise is important. Exercise affects how quickly the body uses food. Exercise also improves circulation. Exercise may include walking or other activities. It may also include passive range of motion exercises. Help with exercises as necessary. Be positive. Try to make it fun.

G   Observe the client's management of insulin. Doses are calculated exactly. They should be administered at the same time each day.

Home health aides are not permitted to inject insulin. However, make sure you know when clients take insulin and when their meals should be served. There must be a balance between the insulin level and food intake.

G   Perform urine and blood tests as directed. Sometimes the care plan will specify a daily blood or urine test for insulin levels. Not all states allow HHAs to do this. Know your state's rules. Your agency will provide training if you are allowed to do these tests.

G   Give foot care as directed. People with diabetes have poor circulation. Even a small sore on the leg or foot can grow into a large wound that may not heal. This can result in amputation. Careful foot care, including regular, daily inspection, is vital. The goals of diabetic foot care are to check for signs of irritation or sores, to promote blood circulation, and to prevent infection.

G   Encourage diabetic clients to wear comfortable, well-fitting leather shoes that do not hurt their feet. Leather shoes breathe and help prevent buildup of moisture. To avoid injuries to the feet, diabetics should never go barefoot. Cotton socks are best to absorb sweat. HHAs should not trim or clip any client's toenails. Only a nurse or doctor should do this.

Providing foot care for the diabetic client

Equipment: basin, bath thermometer, mild soap, washcloth, 2 towels, lotion, cotton socks, shoes or slippers, gloves

1. Wash your hands.

2. Explain the procedure to the client, speaking clearly, slowly, and directly. Maintain face-to-face contact whenever possible.

3. Provide privacy for the client.

4. Fill the basin halfway with warm water. Test water temperature with thermometer or against the inside of your wrist. Ensure it is safe. Water temperature should be no higher than 105°F. Have client check water temperature. Adjust if necessary.

5. Place basin on a bath towel on the floor (if the client is sitting in a chair) or at the foot of the bed (if the client is in bed). Make sure basin is in a position that is comfortable for the client. Support the foot and ankle throughout the procedure.

6. Put on gloves.

7. Remove the client's socks, and completely submerge the client's feet in the water. Soak the feet for 10 to 20 minutes.

8. Put soap on a wet washcloth. Remove one foot from the water. Wash the entire foot gently, including between the toes and around nail beds.

9. Rinse the entire foot, including between the toes.

10. Using a towel, pat the foot dry gently, including between the toes.

11. Repeat steps 8 through 10 for other foot.

12. Starting at the toes and working up to the ankles, gently rub lotion into the feet with circular strokes. Your goal is to increase circulation, so take several minutes on each foot. Do not put lotion between the toes.

13. Observe the feet, ankles, and legs for dry skin, irritation, blisters, redness, sores, corns, discoloration, or swelling.

14. Help client put on socks and shoes or slippers.

15. Put used linens in the laundry. Pour water into the toilet and flush it. Rinse and dry basin. Store basin and supplies.

16. Remove and discard gloves.

17. Wash your hands.

18. Document the procedure, including any abnormalities you observed on the feet, ankles, or legs.

People with diabetes must be very careful about what they eat. To keep their blood glucose levels near normal, they must eat the right amount of the right type of food at the right time. *Special Diets* in Section VI contains more information.

CVA or Stroke

The medical term for a stroke is a cerebrovascular accident (CVA). CVA, or stroke, occurs when blood supply to a part of the brain is blocked or a blood vessel leaks or ruptures within the brain. An ischemic stroke is the most common type of stroke. With this type, the blood supply is blocked. Without blood, part of the brain does not receive oxygen. Brain cells begin to die. Additional damage can occur due to leaking blood, clots, and swelling of the tissues. Warning signs that a stroke is occurring are located in *Medical Emergencies* in Section II.

Strokes can be mild or severe. After a stroke, a person may experience any of these problems:

- Paralysis on one side of the body, called **hemiplegia**
- Weakness on one side of the body, called **hemiparesis**
- Trouble communicating thoughts through speech or writing, called **expressive aphasia**
- Difficulty understanding spoken or written words, called **receptive aphasia**
- Loss of sensations such as temperature or touch
- Loss of bowel or bladder control (incontinence)
- Confusion
- Poor judgment
- Memory loss

- Loss of cognitive abilities
- Tendency to ignore one side of the body, called *one-sided neglect*
- Laughing or crying without any reason, or when it is inappropriate, called **emotional lability**
- Difficulty swallowing, called **dysphagia**

Each side of the brain controls different functions. Symptoms that a person has depend on which side of the brain is affected by the CVA. Weaknesses on the right side of the body indicate that the left side of the brain was affected. Weaknesses on the left side of the body indicate that the right side of the brain was affected.

If the stroke was mild, the client may experience few, if any, complications. Physical therapy may help restore physical abilities. Speech and occupational therapy can also help with communication and performing ADLs.

Guidelines: CVA/Stroke

G Clients with paralysis, weakness, or loss of movement will usually receive physical or occupational therapy. Range of motion exercises will help strengthen muscles and keep joints mobile. Clients may also need to perform leg exercises to aid circulation. Safety is always important when clients are exercising. Assist carefully with exercises as ordered.

G Never refer to the weaker side as the "bad side," or talk about the "bad" leg or arm. The terms *weaker*, *affected*, or *involved* should be used to refer to the side with paralysis.

G Clients with speech loss or communication problems may receive speech therapy. You may be asked to help. This includes helping clients to recognize written words or spoken words. Speech therapists will also evaluate a client's swallowing ability. They will decide if swallowing therapy or thickened liquids are needed.

G Experiencing confusion or memory loss is upsetting. People often cry for no apparent reason after suffering a stroke. Be patient and understanding. Keeping a routine may help clients feel more secure.

G Encourage independence and self-esteem. Let the client do things for himself whenever possible, even if you could do a better or faster job. Make tasks less difficult for the client to do. Acknowledge clients' efforts to do things for themselves even when they are unsuccessful. Praise even the smallest successes to build confidence.

G   Always check on the client's body alignment. Sometimes an arm or leg can be caught and the client is unaware.

G   Pay special attention to skin care and observe for changes in the skin if a client is unable to move.

G   If clients have a loss of touch or sensation, check for potentially harmful situations (for example, heat and sharp objects). If clients are unable to sense or move part of the body, check and change positioning to prevent pressure ulcers.

G   Adapt procedures when caring for clients with one-sided paralysis or weakness. Carefully assist with shaving, grooming, and bathing.

G   When helping with transfers or walking, always use a gait belt for safety. Stand on the weaker side. Support the weaker side and lead with the stronger side.

When assisting with dressing, remember to do the following:

G   Dress the weaker side first. Place the weaker arm or leg into the clothing first. This prevents unnecessary bending and stretching of the limb. Undress the stronger side first. Then remove the weaker arm or leg from clothing to prevent the limb from being stretched and twisted.

G   Use assistive equipment to help the client dress himself. Encourage self-care.

When assisting with communication, remember to do the following:

G   Keep your questions and directions simple.

G   Phrase questions so they can be answered with a "yes" or "no."

G   Agree on signals, such as shaking or nodding the head, or raising a hand or finger to indicate "yes" or "no."

G   Give clients time to respond. Listen attentively.

G   Use a pencil and paper if a client can write. A thick handle or tape around the pencil may help the client hold it more easily.

G   Use verbal and nonverbal communication to express your positive attitude. Let the client know you have confidence in his or her abilities through smiles, touches, and gestures. Gestures and pointing can also help give information or allow the client to communicate.

G   Use communication boards or special cards to aid communication.

G   Keep a bell or other call signal within reach of clients. They can let you know when you are needed.

G   Never talk about a client as if he or she were not there. Speak to all clients with respect.

When assisting with eating, remember to do the following:

G   Place food in the client's field of vision. A nurse or doctor will determine a client's field of vision.

G   Use assistive devices such as silverware with built-up handle grips, plate guards, and drinking cups as needed.

G   Watch for signs of choking.

G   Serve soft foods if swallowing is difficult.

G   Always place food in the unaffected, or stronger, side of the mouth. Make sure food is swallowed before offering more bites.

Monitoring the home safety of clients who have had a stroke is essential. Clients who are unsteady, weak, or confused are at risk of falling. Clients with loss of sensation are at risk of burning themselves in the bathroom or at the stove. Some safety tips include the following:

•   Remove any hazards from the home, including unnecessary clutter or throw rugs.

•   Unplug appliances like toasters and coffee makers when not in use.

•   Check the refrigerator and cabinets for spoiled food. A stroke may impair a person's sense of smell and taste.

•   Report any suspected safety hazards to the supervisor.

Multiple Sclerosis (MS)

Multiple sclerosis (MS) is a progressive disease that affects the central nervous system. When a person has MS, the protective covering for the nerves, spinal cord, and white matter of the brain breaks down over time. Without this covering, or sheath, nerves cannot send messages to and from the brain in a normal way. MS progresses slowly and unpredictably. Clients who have this disease will have widely varying abilities. Symptoms include blurred vision, fatigue, tremors, poor balance, and trouble walking. Weakness, numbness, tingling, incontinence, and behavior changes are also symptoms. MS can cause blindness, contractures, and loss of function in the arms and legs. The exact cause of multiple sclerosis is not known, but it may be an autoimmune disease. There is no cure for this disease; it is mostly treated with medication.

Guidelines: Multiple Sclerosis

G   Assist with ADLs as needed. Be patient with self-care and movement. Allow enough time for tasks. Offer rest periods as necessary.

G   Give client plenty of time to communicate. People with MS may have trouble forming their thoughts. Be patient and do not rush them.

G   Prevent falls, which may be due to a lack of coordination, fatigue, or vision problems.

G   Stress can worsen the effects of MS. Be calm. Listen to clients when they want to talk.

G   Encourage a healthy diet with plenty of fluids.

G   Give regular skin care to prevent pressure ulcers.

G   Assist with range of motion exercises to prevent contractures and to strengthen muscles.

Circulatory Disorders

Hypertension (HTN) or High Blood Pressure

When blood pressure is consistently 140/90 or higher, a person is diagnosed as having **hypertension** (**HTN**), or high blood pressure. Hypertension may be caused by a hardening and narrowing of the blood vessels. It can also result from kidney disease, tumors of the adrenal gland, pregnancy, and certain medications.

Hypertension can develop in people of any age. Signs and symptoms of hypertension are not always obvious, especially in the early stages. Often it is only discovered when a blood pressure measurement is taken. Persons may complain of headache, blurred vision, and dizziness.

Guidelines: Hypertension

G   Hypertension can lead to serious problems such as CVA, heart attack, kidney disease, or blindness. Treatment to control it is vital. Clients may take medication that lowers blood pressure or cholesterol. They may take diuretics. Diuretics are a type of medication that reduce fluid in the body. Offer trips to the bathroom regularly.

G   Clients may also have a prescribed exercise program or a special low-fat, low-sodium diet. Encourage clients to follow their diets and exercise programs.

Coronary Artery Disease (CAD)

Coronary artery disease occurs when the blood vessels in the coronary arteries narrow. This reduces the supply of blood to the heart muscle and deprives it of oxygen and nutrients. Over time, as fatty deposits block the artery, the muscle that was supplied by the blood vessel dies. CAD can lead to heart attack or stroke.

The heart muscle that is not getting enough oxygen causes chest pain, pressure, or discomfort, called **angina pectoris**. The heart needs more oxygen during exercise, stress, excitement, or to digest a heavy meal. In CAD, narrow blood vessels prevent the extra blood with oxygen from getting to the heart.

The pain of angina pectoris is usually described as pressure or tightness in the left side or in the center of the chest, behind the sternum or breastbone. Some people have pain moving down the inside of the left arm or to the neck and left side of the jaw. A person suffering from angina pectoris may perspire or look pale. The person may feel dizzy and have trouble breathing.

Guidelines: Angina Pectoris

G   Rest is extremely important. Rest reduces the heart's need for extra oxygen. It helps the blood flow return to normal, often within three to 15 minutes. Encourage clients to rest.

G   Medication is also needed to relax the walls of the coronary arteries. This allows them to open to get more blood to the heart. This medication, nitroglycerin, is a small tablet that the client places under the tongue, where it dissolves and is rapidly absorbed. Clients who have angina pectoris may keep nitroglycerin on hand to use as symptoms arise. Home health aides are not allowed to give medications. Tell your supervisor if the client needs help taking the medication. Nitroglycerin is also available as a patch. Do not remove the patch. Tell your supervisor immediately if the patch comes off. Nitroglycerin may also come in the form of a spray that the client sprays onto or under the tongue.

G   Clients may also need to avoid heavy meals, overeating, intense exercise, and cold or hot and humid weather.

Myocardial Infarction (MI) or Heart Attack

When blood flow to the heart muscle is blocked, oxygen and nutrients fail to reach the cells in that region. Waste products are not removed, and the muscle cells die. This is called a myocardial infarction (MI) or heart attack. *Medical Emergencies* in Section II contains information on warning signs of an MI.

Guidelines: Myocardial Infarction

G   Most clients who have had an MI will be placed on a regular exercise program. Encourage clients to follow their exercise programs.

G   Clients may be on a diet that is low in fat and cholesterol and/or low in sodium. Encourage clients to follow their special diets.

G Medications may be prescribed to regulate heart rate and blood pressure. If assigned, observe clients taking their medications.

G Quitting smoking will be encouraged. Be supportive.

G A stress management program may be started to help reduce stress levels. Help clients avoid stress and listen if they want to talk.

G Clients recovering from an MI may need to avoid cold temperatures.

Congestive Heart Failure (CHF)

Coronary artery disease, myocardial infarction, hypertension, or other disorders may all damage the heart. When the left side of the heart is affected, blood backs up into the lungs. When the right side of the heart is affected, blood backs up into the legs, feet, or abdomen. When one or both sides of the heart stop pumping blood properly, it is called **congestive heart failure** (**CHF**).

Guidelines: Congestive Heart Failure

G Although CHF is a serious illness, it can be treated and controlled. Medications can strengthen the heart muscle and improve its pumping. If assigned, observe clients taking their medications.

G Medications help remove excess fluids. This means more trips to the bathroom. Assist clients as needed.

G A low-sodium diet or fluid restrictions may be prescribed. Encourage clients to follow diet orders or restrictions.

G A weakened heart may make it hard for clients to walk, carry items, or climb stairs. Limited activity or bedrest may be prescribed. Allow for a period of rest after an activity.

G Measure intake and output of fluids as ordered.

G Clients may be weighed daily at the same time to note weight gain from fluid retention. Weigh clients as instructed.

G Apply elastic leg stockings as ordered to reduce swelling in feet and ankles.

G Range of motion exercises improve muscle tone when activity and exercise are limited. Assist with ROM exercises.

G Extra pillows may help clients who have trouble breathing. Keeping the head of the bed elevated may also help with breathing.

G Assist with personal care and ADLs as needed.

G Some medications that are used to treat CHF (diuretics) may cause low potassium levels in the body, which can cause dizziness.

High-potassium foods and drinks such as winter squash, baked sweet or regular potatoes, beans, raisins, apricots, prunes, bananas, prune juice, and orange juice can help this.

G   Report any of these to your supervisor:

- Trouble breathing; coughing or gurgling with breathing
- Dizziness, confusion, and fainting
- Pale or blue skin
- Low blood pressure
- Swelling of the feet and ankles (edema)
- Bulging veins in the neck
- Weight gain

For cases of poor circulation to the legs and feet, elastic stockings are ordered. These stockings help prevent swelling and blood clots and aid circulation. Elastic stockings are also known as *anti-embolic stockings* or *TED hose.* Elastic stockings may either be knee-high or thigh-high. They need to be put on in the morning, before the client gets out of bed. Legs are at their smallest size then. They are usually removed in the evening.

Putting elastic stockings on a client

Equipment: elastic stockings

1. **Wash your hands.**

2. **Explain the procedure to the client, speaking clearly, slowly, and directly. Maintain face-to-face contact whenever possible.**

3. **Provide privacy for the client.**

4. **The client should be in the supine position (on her back) in bed. With client lying down, remove her socks, shoes, or slippers, and expose one leg. Expose no more than one leg at a time.**

5. **Turn stocking inside out at least to heel area (Fig. 5-1).**

6. **Gently place foot of stocking over toes, foot, and heel (Fig. 5-2). Make sure the heel is in the right place (heel of foot should be in heel of stocking).**

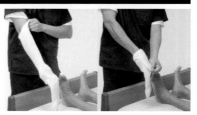

Fig. 5-1. Turning the stocking inside out allows stocking to roll on gently.

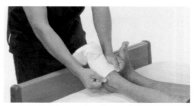

Fig. 5-2. Place the foot of the stocking over the toes, foot, and heel. Promote the client's comfort and safety. Avoid force and over-extension of joints.

7. Gently pull top of stocking over foot, heel, and leg.

8. Make sure there are no twists or wrinkles in stocking after it is on (Fig. 5-3). It must fit smoothly and be comfortable. Make sure the heel of stocking is over the heel of foot. If the stocking has an opening in the toe area, make sure the opening is either over or under the toe area. This depends on the manufacturer's instructions. Adjust if needed.

9. Repeat for other leg.

10. Wash your hands.

11. Document the procedure and your observations. How did the skin appear? Were there any changes in color or temperature? Were there any sores or swelling on the legs?

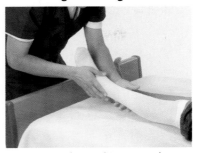

Fig. 5-3. *Make stocking smooth. Twists or wrinkles cause the stocking to be too tight, which reduces circulation.*

HIV and AIDS

Acquired immune deficiency syndrome (AIDS) is a disease caused by the human immunodeficiency virus (HIV). HIV attacks the body's immune system and gradually weakens and disables it. AIDS is the final stage of HIV infection in which infections, tumors, and symptoms appear due to a weakened immune system that is unable to fight infection. It can take years for HIV to develop into AIDS.

HIV is a sexually transmitted disease. It is also spread through blood, from infected needles, or from mother to fetus.

In general, HIV affects the body in stages. The first stage involves symptoms similar to the flu, with fever, muscle aches, cough, and fatigue. These are signs of the immune system fighting the infection. As the infection worsens, the immune system overreacts. It attacks not only the virus, but also normal tissue.

When the virus weakens the immune system in later stages, a group of problems may appear. These include infections, tumors, and central nervous system symptoms. These problems would not occur if the immune system were healthy. This stage of the disease is known as AIDS. The diagnosis of AIDS is made when a person's CD4+ lymphocyte (a type of white blood cell) count falls to 200 or below. In the late stages of AIDS, damage to the central nervous system may cause memory loss, poor coordination, paralysis, and confusion. These symptoms together are known as AIDS dementia complex.

The following are the signs and symptoms of HIV infection and AIDS:

- Flu-like symptoms, including fever, cough, weakness, and severe or constant fatigue
- Appetite loss
- Weight loss
- Night sweats
- Swollen lymph nodes in the neck, underarms, or groin
- Severe diarrhea
- Dry cough
- Skin rashes
- Painful white spots in the mouth or on the tongue
- Cold sores or fever blisters on the lips and flat, white ulcers in the mouth
- Cauliflower-like warts on the skin and in the mouth
- Inflamed and bleeding gums
- Bruising that does not go away
- Low resistance to infection, particularly pneumonia, but also tuberculosis, herpes, bacterial infections, and hepatitis
- Kaposi's sarcoma, a form of skin cancer that appears as purple or red skin lesions
- Pneumocystis pneumonia, a lung infection
- AIDS dementia complex

Infections, such as pneumonia, tuberculosis, or hepatitis, invade the body when the immune system is weak and cannot defend itself. These illnesses worsen AIDS. They further weaken the immune system. It is difficult to treat these infections. Over time, a person may develop a resistance to some antibiotics. These infections often cause death in people with AIDS.

There is no cure for this disease, and there is no vaccine to prevent the disease. People who are infected with HIV are treated with drugs that slow the progress of the disease. Without medication, however, a weakened resistance to infections may lead to AIDS and eventually to death.

A combination of medications can help people with HIV live longer. The medicines must be taken at precise times. They have many unpleasant side effects. For some people, the medications work less well than for others. Other aspects of HIV treatment include relief of symptoms and prevention of infection.

Guidelines: HIV and AIDS

G   People with poor immune system function are more sensitive to infections. Wash your hands often and keep everything clean. Follow Standard Precautions.

G   Involuntary weight loss occurs in almost all people who develop AIDS. High-protein, high-calorie, and high-nutrient meals and supplements can help maintain a healthy weight.

G   Some people with HIV/AIDS lose their appetites and have trouble eating. Serve familiar and favorite foods in a pleasant setting. Report appetite loss or trouble eating to your supervisor.

G   Carefully follow guidelines for safe food preparation and storage when working with a client who has HIV/AIDS. Foodborne illnesses caused by improperly cooking or storing food can cause death for someone with HIV/AIDS. Wash your hands frequently. Keep everything clean, especially countertops, cutting boards, and knives after they have been used to cut meat. Thaw food in the refrigerator, and wash and cook foods thoroughly. When storing food, keep cold foods cold and hot foods hot. Use small containers that seal tightly. Check expiration dates, and remember, "when in doubt, throw it out."

G   Clients who have infections of the mouth may need food that is low in acid and neither cold nor hot. Spicy seasonings should not be used. Soft or pureed foods may be easier to swallow. Liquid meals and fortified drinks, such as milkshakes, may ease the pain of chewing. Warm rinses may help painful mouth sores. Careful mouth care is vital.

G   A person who has nausea or vomiting should eat small, frequent meals and should eat slowly. The person should avoid high-fat and spicy foods and eat a soft, bland diet. This includes mashed potatoes, noodles, rice, crackers, pretzels, toast, gelatin, and clear soups. Cold foods that have little odor are usually easier to eat than hot foods. When nausea and vomiting persist, liquids and salty foods should be encouraged. These include clear soups, clear juices, ginger ale, saltines, and pretzels. Clients should drink fluids in between meals. Proper intake of fluids to balance lost fluids is important.

G   Clients who have mild diarrhea may have small, frequent meals that are low in fat, fiber, and milk products. If diarrhea is severe, the doctor may order a BRAT diet (a diet of bananas, rice, applesauce, and toast). This diet is helpful for short-term use. Diarrhea rapidly depletes the body of fluids. Fluid replacement is necessary. Good rehydration fluids include water, juice, caffeine-free soda, and broth. Caffeinated drinks should be avoided.

G **Neuropathy**, or numbness, tingling, and pain in the feet and legs is usually treated with medications. Wearing loose, soft slippers may be helpful. If blankets cause pain, use a bed cradle to keep sheets and blankets from resting on the legs and feet.

G Give emotional support, as well as physical care. Clients with HIV/AIDS may suffer from anxiety and depression. In addition, they are often judged by family, friends, and society. Some people blame them for their illness. People with HIV/AIDS may feel tremendous stress. They may be uncertain about their illness, health care, and finances. They may also have lost friends who have died from AIDS. Treat clients with respect. Help give the emotional support they need. Clients with this disease need support from others. This may come from family, friends, religious and community groups, and support groups, as well as the care team.

G Withdrawal, avoidance of tasks, and mental slowness are early symptoms of HIV. Medications may also cause side effects of this type. AIDS dementia complex may cause further mental symptoms. There may also be muscle weakness and loss of muscle control, making falls a risk. Clients will need a safe environment and close supervision in their ADLs.

Dementia

As a person ages, some of the ability to think logically and quickly may be lost. This ability is called cognition. When some of this ability is lost, a person is said to have *cognitive impairment*. How much ability is lost depends on the individual. Cognitive impairment affects concentration and memory. Elderly clients may lose their memories of recent events, which can be frustrating for them. HHAs can help by encouraging them to make lists of things to remember. Writing down names, events, and phone numbers may also help. Other normal changes of aging in the brain include slower reaction time, trouble finding or using the right words, and sleeping less.

Dementia is a general term that refers to a serious loss of mental abilities such as thinking, remembering, reasoning, and communicating. As dementia advances, these losses make it difficult to perform activities of daily living (ADLs) such as eating, bathing, dressing, and toileting. Dementia is not a normal part of aging.

These are some common causes of dementia:

• Alzheimer's disease

• Multi-infarct dementia or vascular dementia (a series of strokes that cause damage to the brain)

- Lewy body dementia (abnormal structures, called Lewy bodies, develop in areas of the brain, causing a variety of symptoms)
- Parkinson's disease
- Huntington's disease (an inherited disease that causes certain nerve cells in the brain to waste away)

Alzheimer's Disease (AD)

Alzheimer's disease (AD) is the most common cause of dementia in the elderly. This disease causes tangled nerve fibers and protein deposits to form in the brain, eventually causing dementia. The disease gets worse, causing greater and greater loss of health and abilities. There is no known cause of Alzheimer's disease and there is no cure. Clients with Alzheimer's disease will never recover. They will need more care as the disease progresses.

Symptoms of AD appear gradually. It begins with memory loss. As AD progresses, the symptoms get worse. The disease progresses to complete loss of all ability to care for oneself. Each person with AD will show different symptoms at different times. For example, one client with AD may continue to read, but not be able to use the phone. Another person may lose the ability to read, but can still do simple math. Skills a person has used over a lifetime are usually kept longer.

It is important for HHAs to encourage independence, regardless of what signs a person with AD shows. Clients with AD should be encouraged to do their ADLs. This helps keep their minds and bodies as active as possible. Socializing, reading, problem solving, and exercising should all be encouraged. Having clients do as much as possible for themselves may even help slow the progression of the disease. Tasks should be challenging but not frustrating. HHAs can help clients succeed in doing these tasks.

These tips help home health aides give the best possible care to clients with Alzheimer's disease:

- Do not take things personally.
- Be empathetic.
- Work with the symptoms and behaviors noted.
- Work as a team.
- Be aware of difficulties associated with caregiving.
- Work with family members.
- Remember the goals of the care plan.

Guidelines: Communicating with Clients Who Have Alzheimer's Disease

G   Always approach from the front. Do not startle the client.

G   Determine how close the client wants you to be.

G   Speak in a low, calm voice, in a room with little background noise and distraction.

G   Always identify yourself and use the client's name. Continue to use the client's name during the conversation.

G   Speak slowly, using a lower tone of voice than normal.

G   Repeat yourself, using the same words and phrases as often as needed.

G   Use signs, pictures, gestures, or written words to help communicate.

G   Break complex tasks into smaller, simpler ones. Give simple, step-by-step instructions as necessary.

Home health aides should use the same procedures for personal care and ADLs for clients with Alzheimer's disease as they would with other clients. However, there are some general principles that will help give the best care:

1.   Develop a routine and stick to it. Being consistent is very important for clients who are confused and easily upset.

2.   Promote self-care. Helping clients care for themselves as much as possible will help them cope with this difficult disease.

3.   HHAs should take good care of themselves, both mentally and physically. This will help them give the best possible care.

Guidelines: Caring for Clients with Alzheimer's Disease

G   Schedule bathing when the client is least agitated. Be organized so the bath can be quick.

G   Be flexible about bathing. A client may not always be in the mood. Be relaxed. Allow the client to enjoy the bath. Check the skin regularly when bathing for signs of irritation.

G   Ensure safety by using non-slip mats, tub seats, and hand-holds.

G   Assist with grooming to help clients feel attractive and dignified.

G   Lay out clothes in the order in which they should be put on. Choose clothes that are simple to put on.

G   Encourage fluids. Never withhold or discourage fluids because a person is incontinent. Follow schedules for toileting.

G Mark the bathroom with a sign or a picture to remind the client where it is and to use the toilet.

G Put lids on trash cans, wastebaskets, or other containers if the client urinates in them.

G Schedule meals at the same time each day. Serve familiar, appetizing foods. Try smaller, more frequent meals if person is restless. Finger foods can allow eating while moving around. Keep bite-sized snacks nearby, especially favorites.

G Do not serve steaming or very hot foods or drinks. Use a simple place setting with a single eating utensil, and remove other items from the table. Plain plates without patterns or colors work best. Put only one item of food on the plate at a time.

G Guide the client through meals. Provide simple instructions. Offer regular drinks of water, juice, and other fluids to avoid dehydration. Make mealtime simple and relaxed.

G Prevent infections. Follow proper procedures for food preparation and storage, household management, and Standard Precautions.

G Observe the client's physical health and report any potential problems.

G Give careful skin care to prevent pressure ulcers.

G Watch for signs of pain.

G Maintain a daily exercise routine.

G Maintain self-esteem by encouraging independence in ADLs.

G Share in enjoyable activities, looking at pictures, talking, and reminiscing.

G Reward positive and independent behavior with smiles, warm touches, and thanks.

Below are some common difficult behaviors that HHAs may face when working with clients with Alzheimer's disease:

Agitation: Try to remove triggers, keep a routine, and avoid frustration. Help client focus on a soothing, familiar activity, such as sorting things or looking at pictures. Remain calm. Use a low, soothing voice to speak to and reassure the client. An arm around the shoulder or patting the client may be soothing.

Sundowning: When a person becomes restless and agitated in the late afternoon, evening, or night, it is called **sundowning**. Remove triggers, give snacks, and encourage rest. Avoid stressful situations during this time. Limit activities, appointments, trips, and visits. Play soft music.

Set a bedtime routine and keep it. Recognize when sundowning occurs and plan a calming activity just before. Remove caffeine from the diet. Give a soothing back massage. Distract the client with a simple, calm activity like looking at a magazine. Maintain a daily exercise routine.

Catastrophic Reactions: When a person with AD overreacts to something, it is called a catastrophic reaction. A catastrophic reaction may be triggered by fatigue; a change of routine, environment, or caregiver; overstimulation; difficult choices or tasks; physical pain; hunger; or a need for toileting. For these reactions, remove triggers and help the client focus on a soothing activity.

Violent Behavior: A client who attacks, hits, or threatens someone is violent. Frustration, overstimulation, or a change in routine, environment, or caregiver may trigger violence. For violent clients, block blows, but never hit back. Step out of reach. Call for help if needed. Avoid leaving the client in the home alone. Try to remove triggers. Use the same techniques to calm client as for agitation or sundowning.

Pacing and Wandering: A client who walks back and forth in the same area is pacing. A client who walks aimlessly around the house or neighborhood is wandering. Pacing and wandering may be caused by restlessness, hunger, disorientation, need for toileting, constipation, pain, forgetting how or where to sit down, too much daytime napping, or the need for exercise. Remove causes when you can. For example, give nutritious snacks and maintain a toileting schedule. Let clients pace and wander in a safe and secure (locked) area where they can be watched. Suggest another activity, such as going for a walk together.

Hallucinations or Delusions: A person who sees, hears, smells, tastes, or feels things that are not there is having hallucinations. A person who believes things that are not true is having delusions. Ignore harmless hallucinations and delusions. Reassure a client who seems agitated or worried. Do not argue with a client who is imagining things. Do not tell the client that you can see or hear his hallucinations. Redirect the client to other activities or thoughts. Be calm and reassure the client that you are there to help.

Depression: Report signs of depression to your supervisor immediately. It is an illness that can be treated with medication and therapy. Encourage independence, self-care, and activity. Talk about moods and feelings if the client wishes. Be a good listener. Encourage social interaction.

Perseveration or Repetitive Phrasing: A client who repeats a word, phrase, question, or activity over and over is **perseverating**. This may be caused by disorientation or confusion. Respond to perseveration with patience. Do not try to silence or stop the client. Answer questions each time they are asked, using the same words each time.

Disruptiveness: Disruptive behavior is anything that disturbs others, such as yelling, banging on furniture, slamming doors, etc. Often this behavior is triggered by a wish for attention, by pain or constipation, or by frustration. When this behavior happens, gain the client's attention. Be calm and friendly. Try to find out why the behavior is happening. To try to prevent this behavior, notice and praise improvements in the client's behavior. Be sensitive when you do this to avoid treating the client like a child. Tell the client about any changes in schedules, routines, or the environment in advance. Involve the client in developing routine activities and schedules. Encourage the client to join in independent activities that are safe (for example, folding towels). This can prevent feelings of powerlessness. Help the client find ways to cope. Focus on positive activities he may still be able to do, such as knitting or crafts.

Inappropriate Social Behavior: Inappropriate social behavior may be cursing, name calling, or other behavior. As with violent or disruptive behavior, there may be many reasons why a client is behaving this way. Try not to take it personally. The client may only be reacting to frustration or other stress. Stay calm and be reassuring. Try to find out what caused the behavior (such as too much noise, too many people, too much stress, pain, or discomfort). Respond positively to any appropriate behavior. Any physical abuse or serious verbal abuse should be reported.

Inappropriate Sexual Behavior: Inappropriate sexual behavior, such as removing clothes, touching one's own genitals, or trying to touch others can embarrass those who see it. Do not overreact when dealing with this behavior. This may reinforce the behavior. Be sensitive to the nature of the problem. Try to distract the client. A client may be reacting to a need for physical stimulation or affection. Ways to provide physical stimulation include backrubs, a soft doll or stuffed animal to cuddle, comforting blankets, or physical touch that is appropriate.

Sleep Disturbances: Clients with AD may experience a number of sleep disturbances. Make sure the client gets moderate exercise/activity throughout the day. Encourage him to participate in activities he enjoys. Allow the client to spend some time each day in natural sunlight if possible. Exposure to light and dark can help establish restful sleep patterns. Reduce light and noise as much as possible during nighttime hours. Discourage sleeping during the day.

Although Alzheimer's disease cannot be cured, there are techniques that can improve the quality of life for clients with AD.

Reality orientation involves the use of calendars, clocks, signs, and lists to help clients remember who and where they are. It is useful in the early stages of Alzheimer's disease when clients are confused but not totally disoriented. In later stages, reality orientation may only frustrate clients.

Validation therapy is letting clients believe they live in the past or in imaginary circumstances. **Validating** means giving value to or approving. Make no attempt to reorient clients to actual circumstances. Explore clients' beliefs and do not argue with or correct them. It is useful in cases of moderate to severe disorientation.

Reminiscence therapy is encouraging clients to remember and talk about the past. Explore memories by asking about details. Focus on a time of life that was pleasant. Work through feelings about a difficult time in the past. It is useful in many stages of Alzheimer's disease, but especially with moderate to severe confusion.

Activity therapy uses activities clients enjoy to prevent boredom and frustration. These activities also promote self-esteem. Help clients to take walks, do puzzles, listen to music, cook, read, or do other activities they enjoy. It is useful throughout most stages of Alzheimer's disease.

Chronic Obstructive Pulmonary Disease (COPD)

Chronic obstructive pulmonary disease (COPD) is a chronic disease. This means the client may live for years with it but never be cured. Clients with COPD have difficulty breathing, especially in getting air out of the lungs. There are two chronic lung diseases that are grouped under COPD: chronic bronchitis and emphysema.

Over time, a client with either of these lung disorders becomes chronically ill and weakened. There is a high risk for acute lung infections, such as pneumonia. When the lungs and brain do not get enough oxygen, all body systems are affected. Clients may live with a constant fear of not being able to breathe. This can cause them to sit upright in an attempt to improve their ability to expand the lungs. These clients can have poor appetites. They usually do not get enough sleep. All of this can add to their feelings of weakness and poor health. They may feel they have lost control of their bodies, particularly their breathing. They may fear suffocation.

Clients with COPD may experience the following symptoms:

- Chronic cough or wheeze
- Trouble breathing, especially with inhaling and exhaling deeply
- Shortness of breath, especially during physical exertion

- Pale, blue (cyanotic), reddish-purple skin
- Confusion
- General state of weakness
- Trouble completing meals due to shortness of breath
- Fear and anxiety

Guidelines: Chronic Obstructive Pulmonary Disease

G   Colds or viruses can quickly make clients very ill. Always observe and report signs of symptoms getting worse.

G   Help clients sit upright or lean forward. Offer pillows for support.

G   Offer plenty of fluids and small, frequent meals.

G   Encourage a well-balanced diet.

G   Keep oxygen supply available as ordered.

G   Being unable to breathe or fearing suffocation can be very frightening. Be calm and supportive.

G   Use infection prevention practices. Wash your hands often and encourage the client to do the same. Dispose of used tissues promptly.

G   Encourage as much independence with ADLs as possible.

G   Remind clients to avoid exposure to infections, especially colds and the flu.

G   Encourage pursed-lip breathing. Pursed-lip breathing involves inhaling slowly through the nose and exhaling slowly through pursed lips (as if about to whistle). A nurse should teach clients how to do this.

G   Encourage clients to save energy for important tasks. Encourage clients to rest.

Tuberculosis (TB)

Tuberculosis, or TB, is a highly contagious lung disease. It is caused by a bacterium that is carried on mucous droplets suspended in the air. When a person infected with TB talks, coughs, breathes, sings, laughs, or sneezes, he may release mucous droplets carrying the disease. TB usually infects the lungs, causing coughing, difficulty breathing, fever, weight loss, and fatigue. Usually TB can be cured by taking all of the prescribed medication. However, if left untreated, TB may cause death.

Symptoms of TB include prolonged coughing, pain in the chest, coughing up blood or sputum, fatigue, loss of appetite, weight loss, chills, fever, and night sweats.

When caring for clients who have TB, HHAs should follow Standard Precautions and Airborne Precautions. They should use personal protective equipment as instructed. Special masks, such as N95, high efficiency particulate air (HEPA), or other masks must be used. HHAs must take care when handling sputum and follow isolation procedures if directed. They should help the client remember to take all medication prescribed. Failure to do so is a major factor in the spread of TB. Multidrug-resistant TB (MDR-TB) can develop when people with TB disease do not take all of the prescribed medication.

Hip or Knee Replacement

Total hip replacement (THR) is the surgical replacement of the head of the long bone of the leg (femur) where it joins the hip. This surgery is often done for these reasons:

- Hip is fractured from an injury or fall that does not heal properly.
- Hip is weakened due to aging.
- Hip is painful and stiff because the joint is weak and the bones are no longer strong enough to bear the person's weight.

After the surgery, the client cannot stand on that leg while the area heals. A physical therapist will assist after surgery. The goals of care include slowly strengthening the hip muscles and getting the client to bear weight on that leg. The client's care plan will state when the client may begin to put weight on the leg. It will also give instructions on how much the client is able to do. HHAs should help with personal care and with using assistive devices, such as walkers or canes. Pain monitoring and prevention will be important. HHAs should report to the supervisor any complaints of pain or unrelieved pain.

Guidelines: Hip Replacement

G   Keep often-used items, such as medications, telephone, tissues, call signals, and water, within easy reach. Avoid placing items in high places.

G   Dress the affected (weaker) side first.

G   Never rush the client. Use praise and encouragement often. Do this even for small accomplishments.

G   Have the client sit to do tasks to save her energy.

G   Follow the care plan exactly, even if the client wants to do more. Follow orders for weight-bearing. After surgery, the doctor's order will be written as *partial weight-bearing* (PWB) or *non-weight-bearing*

(*NWB*). Partial weight-bearing means the client is able to support some body weight on one or both legs. Non-weight-bearing means the client is unable to touch the floor or support any weight on one or both legs. Once the client can bear full weight again, the doctor's order will be written for *full weight-bearing* (*FWB*). Full weight-bearing means that both legs can bear 100 percent of the body weight on a step. Help as needed with cane, walker, or crutches.

G Never perform range of motion exercises on the operative leg unless directed by the supervisor.

G Caution the client not to sit with her legs crossed. The hip cannot be bent or flexed more than 90 degrees. It cannot be turned inward or outward.

G An abduction pillow will nor-mally be used for six to 12 weeks after surgery while the client is sleeping in bed. The abduction pillow immobilizes and positions the hips and lower extremities. The pillow is placed in between the legs. The legs are secured to the sides of pillow using straps (Fig. 5-4). If ordered to use this pillow, fol-low instructions for application and positioning.

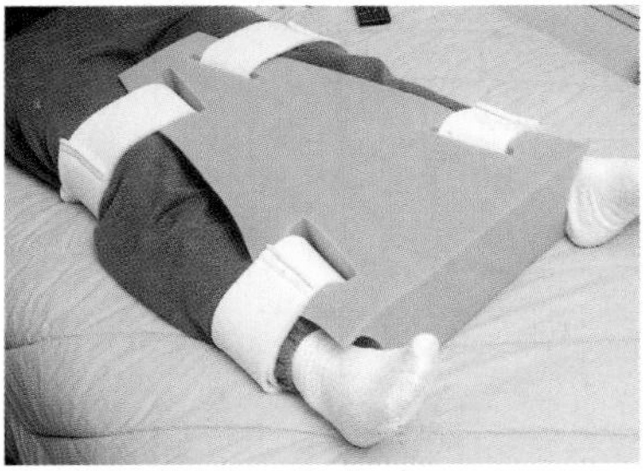

Fig. 5-4. *An abduction pillow is placed in between the legs to immo-bilize and position the hips and lower extremities.* (PHOTO COURTESY OF NORTH COAST MEDICAL, INC., WWW.NCMEDICAL.COM, 800-821-9319)

G When transferring from a bed, use a pillow between the thighs to keep the legs separated. Raise the head of the bed. This allows the client to move her legs over the side of the bed with the thighs still separated. Stand on the side of the unaffected hip. The strong side should lead in standing, pivoting, and sitting.

G With chair or toilet transfers, the operative leg should be straight-ened. The stronger leg should stand first (with a walker or crutches). Then the foot of the affected leg can be brought back to the walking position.

G Report any of the following to your supervisor:

● Redness, drainage, bleeding, or warmth in incision area

● An increase in pain

● Numbness or tingling

● Shortening and/or external rotation of affected leg

- Abnormal vital signs, especially change in temperature
- Client cannot use equipment properly and safely
- Client is not following doctor's orders for activity and exercise
- Any problems with appetite
- Any improvements, such as increased strength and improved ability to walk

Total knee replacement (TKR) is the surgical replacement of the knee with a prosthetic knee. A **prosthesis** is a device that replaces a body part that is missing or deformed because of an accident, injury, illness, or birth defect. It is used to improve a person's ability to function and/or his appearance. This surgery is performed to relieve pain. It also restores motion to a knee damaged by injury or arthritis. It can help stabilize a knee that buckles or gives out repeatedly. Care is similar to that for hip replacement, but the recovery time is much shorter. These clients have more ability to care for themselves. Therefore, they are not seen in home care as often as clients with hip replacements.

Guidelines: Knee Replacement

G   To prevent blood clots, apply special stockings as ordered.

G   Perform ankle pumps as ordered. These are simple exercises that promote circulation to the legs. Ankle pumps are done by raising the toes and feet toward the ceiling and lowering them again.

G   Encourage fluids, especially cranberry and orange juice, which contain vitamin C, to prevent urinary tract infections (UTIs).

G   Assist with deep breathing exercises as ordered.

G   Report to your supervisor if you notice redness, swelling, heat, or deep tenderness in one or both calves.

VI. Home Management and Nutrition

The Client's Environment

Housekeeping

Providing a safe, clean, and orderly environment has always been an essential part of home health care. Clients feel better physically and psychologically and recover more quickly when their homes and families receive care and support. Infection and accidents are prevented. Home health aides can be role models for clients and their families by performing household tasks efficiently and cheerfully.

It takes efficiency, planning, knowledge, and skill to manage a household. An HHA will need to know how to use his time and energy wisely. This is so he does not neglect his primary responsibility—the personal care of the client. Sensitivity is another important quality when caring for clients' homes. HHAs must respect clients' customs, beliefs, and feelings.

Housekeeping assignments will vary. They may include simple cleaning and organizing of the client's room or general cleaning throughout the house. Some clients require management of all household functions, including finances. An HHA may be required to dust, straighten, vacuum, sweep, wash dishes, clean the bathroom and kitchen, and do laundry. The assignments will outline the specific duties to be performed. Most agencies require that HHAs perform light housekeeping. This usually involves dusting, straightening, vacuuming or sweeping floors, cleaning bathrooms and the kitchen, and disposing of trash.

Guidelines: Housekeeping

G   Invite family participation. Depending on their abilities and availability, clients and family members may be asked to participate in housekeeping tasks.

G   Invite family and client input when you determine the tasks that need to be done and the methods used.

G   Use cleaning materials and methods that are acceptable to and approved by clients and their families. Any efforts you make toward improving the home environment should coincide with the client's choices, lifestyle, and values.

G   Be organized when performing tasks. Write out detailed daily and weekly schedules. Seek feedback from your supervisor and the client and family.

G   Build some flexibility into the schedule to allow for changes in the client's condition, needs, appointments, or social activities.

G   Organize cleaning materials and equipment by placing them in one closet. Do not leave cleaning equipment around the home.

G   Familiarize yourself with the household's cleaning materials and equipment. Read the labels and instruction booklets.

G   Maintain a safe environment, as well as a clean one. Do not wax floors if your client is unsteady. Mop up spills immediately.

G   Use housekeeping procedures and methods that promote health.

G   Observe the home for signs of infestation by roaches, rats, mice, lice, and fleas. Some of these insects and animals are common carriers of disease. Report signs of infestation to your supervisor.

G   Use proper body mechanics when performing activities to prevent injury. Watch your posture. Kneel instead of stooping for periods.

G   Clean up and straighten up after every activity. Spills that have dried are difficult to remove later.

G   Carry paper and a small pencil to make note of items that must be purchased or replaced. Maintain a shopping list on a refrigerator door or other convenient location. Encourage family members to use the list.

G   Use your time wisely and efficiently. For example, prepare food while a load of wash is being done.

All cleaning products must be used properly. Many cleaning products are chemicals, which can be irritating and can even cause burns. Some chemicals are poisonous when swallowed.

Guidelines: Using Household Cleaning Products

G   Read and follow the directions on the label of every product you use. Cleaning products can harm the materials and surfaces you are trying to clean.

G   Do not mix cleaning products. This can cause a dangerous chemical reaction that may harm you or others. In particular, never mix bleach or products containing bleach with ammonia. The fumes are toxic and can be fatal.

G   Open windows when cleaning to provide fresh air. Some cleaning products may have fumes that are unpleasant or even harmful if you are exposed to them for a long time.

G   Do not leave cleaning products on surfaces longer than the recommended time. Do not scrub too hard on soft surfaces.

G   Household bleach, diluted with four parts water, makes a strong disinfectant solution to clean bathroom surfaces. Diluted with nine parts water and stored in a spray bottle, bleach makes a milder disinfectant to use on kitchen counters. Do not spill bleach or bleach solutions on carpets, clothing, or other surfaces that might be discolored.

Cleaning Solution Ideas

Several types of environmentally-safe, non-toxic cleaning solutions can be prepared from common household items.

- Baking soda can be used instead of scouring powder. Baking soda can also be diluted with warm water to make a solution that will eliminate odors when used to clean surfaces.

- White vinegar can be used to remove lime or other mineral deposits on sinks, toilets, or chrome fixtures. It cuts grease and removes mildew and odors. White vinegar diluted with water can be used instead of glass cleaner. Mix solution using one part white vinegar to three parts water (1:3). This solution can also be used to clean sealed wood and tile floors.

- Lemon juice, by itself or mixed with water or other ingredients, can be used to eliminate odors, clean and disinfect surfaces, and cut grease.

Not all housekeeping tasks must be performed daily. Some tasks may be done weekly. Others only need to be done once a month or seasonally. The special tasks can be spaced out. Each cleaning job should be done properly and efficiently. Housework can be made safer by not reaching, bending, and stooping unnecessarily. The HHA can experiment to find the most comfortable and effective way to do each job. Cleaning can be done when a client is resting, sleeping, or doing another activity. Care of the client is the HHA's primary responsibility. However, he must not neglect housekeeping.

Guidelines: Straightening and Cleaning Living Areas

G   Clear clutter and put objects in their proper places.

G Pick up newspapers, magazines, and toys as needed.

G Empty wastebaskets and ashtrays daily.

G Make the beds each day.

G Keep essential and frequently-used items, such as eyeglasses, tissues, a wastebasket, telephone, laptop, tablet, newspaper, magazines, and books, within reach.

G Dust once a week or when necessary. If your client has allergies, you may need to dust daily.

G Vacuum floors and rugs once a week or more often if indicated. If the home does not have a vacuum, use a broom to sweep the floors and rugs. Take care not to raise much dust.

G Floors covered with vinyl, ceramic tile, and linoleum may be washed. Some wood floors may not. Some floor coverings should be cleaned with water only. Check with the client or family before you begin. After removing loose dirt or crumbs with a vacuum or broom, wash floors with a cloth or mop dipped in warm sudsy water (or proper cleaning solution). Dry the floor after you have washed it, or close off the area for the time it takes for the floor to dry.

Handling food on contaminated surfaces, improper dishwashing, and contaminated food storage areas may transmit disease. Roaches, rats, and mice may cause disease and allergic reactions by contaminating food with their saliva or their droppings. Pest control is vital to health and cleanliness. An HHA should always report pest control problems to his supervisor.

Guidelines: Cleaning the Kitchen

G Clean the kitchen after every use. Ask family members to do the same. Do not wait until the end of the day to clean up. Daily kitchen cleaning tasks include washing dishes, wiping surfaces, taking out garbage, and storing leftover food. Weekly tasks include cleaning the refrigerator and washing the floor. Cleaning cabinets, drawers, and other storage areas is usually done a few times a year.

G Wash dishes in hot soapy water using liquid dish detergent. Rinse them in hot water. When working with clients who have an infectious disease or a cold, use boiling water for rinsing and add a tablespoon of chlorine bleach to the soapy water. The combination of heat and chlorine will kill pathogens, or harmful microorganisms.

G Wash glasses and cups first, then silverware, plates, and bowls. Pots and pans are washed last. Rinse with hot water and dry on a rack. Air drying dishes is more sanitary than drying with a dish towel.

G   If the house has a dishwasher, learn how to correctly load and start it. Dishwashers save time. They may also sterilize dishes due to the high temperatures used in washing and drying. Use only dishwasher detergent in the dishwasher. Fill the well with only the amount recommended on the label.

G   Do not wash the following items in the dishwasher: electrical appliances, certain plastic materials, wooden pieces or utensils, hand-painted or antique dishes, delicate china, crystal, cast iron, most pots and pans, and sharp or carbon steel knives.

G   Clean the outside of the stove, the trays, and burners with hot, sudsy water or an all-purpose cleaner, and rinse. Ovens should be cleaned according to manufacturer's recommendations.

G   The refrigerator should be completely cleaned once a week. However, you should wipe it out more frequently. If the freezer is not a self-defrosting one, defrost it whenever necessary. To defrost a freezer, turn the dial to the off position. Read the directions on the freezer.

G   Mix two tablespoons of baking soda in one quart of warm water. Wipe the inside walls of the refrigerator and freezer. Baking soda will remove odors. Wash the shelves and trays with warm, soapy water.

G   Clean countertops, tables, and the stove each time they are used. Clean cabinet and drawer fronts once a week. If a cutting board or other surface has been used to cut fresh meat, scrub the surface thoroughly with hot, soapy water. Rinse well.

G   An all-purpose cleaner or a vinegar or lemon juice solution may be needed to remove grease and cooked foods that have spilled or splashed on surfaces. Clean the sink with scouring powder or baking soda.

G   Never place food on soiled work or storage areas or in unclean containers. Keep food covered. Close lids of cartons and cover food storage containers to prevent contamination or infestation by insects and rodents. Place leftovers in covered containers and store them in the refrigerator immediately. Use them within two to three days.

G   Vacuum, sweep, or dry mop the floor daily. Damp mop uncarpeted floors at least once a week, using hot water and a floor cleaner or a vinegar solution. Rinse the floor if label recommends doing so. Dry the floor or close off the area until the floor dries to prevent accidents.

G   Dispose of garbage daily. To prevent odor and discourage insects and rodents, rinse out tin cans and bottles before placing them in the garbage pail or recycling bin. Follow the recycling procedures for your client's community. Periodically wash wastebaskets and trash cans with hot, soapy water.

G   Store all cleaning materials away from food, food preparation utensils, and food preparation areas. Keep them out of reach of children and confused clients.

Recycling

Recycling is the process of taking materials that would have been considered waste and turning them into new products. Recycling programs help reduce waste and the need for landfills. Recycling helps prevent pollution and saves energy, among many other benefits. Some clients will have recycling bins in their homes. Certain plastics, glass, steel, aluminum, and paper products are commonly placed in recycling bins. Other items, such as electronics and batteries, usually need to be recycled separately. Make sure you know which materials can be recycled and how to recycle in your client's community. You may need to rinse recyclable items and sort them into separate bins. If in doubt, ask the client or your supervisor. Use recycling bins as directed.

A clean, organized, and odor-free bathroom is an important part of improving a family's hygiene and safety. Because it is moist and warm, the bathroom is a reservoir for the growth of microorganisms, mold, and mildew.

Guidelines: Cleaning the Bathroom

G   Involve the entire family in keeping the bathroom clean. Always wash from clean areas to dirty areas, so you do not spread dirt into areas that have already been washed.

G   Flush the toilet each time it is used.

G   Clean toothbrushes and toothbrush holders.

G   Scrub the tub and shower after use.

G   Remove hair from drain strainers.

G   Hang up all used towels to dry.

G   Put away toiletries.

G   Rinse the sink after brushing teeth, shaving, and washing.

G   Place soiled towels in the laundry hamper after they are dry.

The bathroom is the location of many home accidents. All bathroom rugs should be nonskid, and puddles of water should be wiped up immediately. If grab bars are not present and a client has difficulty moving about in the bathroom safely, the HHA should report this to his supervisor.

Cleaning the bathroom

Equipment: approved disinfectant (a cleaning product that kills germs), scouring powder or baking soda, floor cleaner or vinegar solution, rags or disposable wipes, toilet brush, glass cleaner or vinegar solution, paper towels, disposable or rubber gloves

1. Put on gloves.

2. Using the disinfectant and rag/wipe, wipe all surfaces and rinse as needed. Be sure to clean the sides, walls, and curtain or door of the shower or tub; the towel racks; holders for toilet paper, toothbrushes, and soap; and window sills.

3. Use a different rag/wipe to wipe the outside of the toilet bowl, seat, and lid. As a general cleaning rule, start with the cleanest surface first, then move to dirtier areas.

4. Use a different rag/wipe to clean the bathtub, shower stall, and sink. Use scouring powder or baking soda for tile and porcelain, and disinfectant or vinegar solution on other surfaces. Remember that scouring powder can scratch. Check with the client or a family member before using it. Be sure to scrub the sides, edges, and bottoms of all these areas. Clean faucets and scrub around their bases.

5. Scrub the inside of the toilet bowl with a toilet brush and scouring powder. Be sure to scrub under the rim. If you use a second, stronger toilet cleaner, flush the first cleaning product first to avoid possible chemical reactions. Wash the toilet brush with a disinfectant solution. Store it in a holder after letting it air dry.

6. Vacuum or dry mop the floor first, then wash if the floor is tile or linoleum. Use an all-purpose floor cleaner or vinegar solution in hot water. Wash the floor with a cloth or mop, taking special care to clean the areas at the base of the toilet and sink. Do not leave the floor wet. Dry it carefully to avoid accidents.

7. Clean the mirror and any glass or chrome surfaces using glass cleaner or vinegar solution and paper towels or clean rags.

8. Launder wet, soiled rags or discard wipes. Empty the waste can into a plastic or paper garbage bag and dispose of the waste. Replace toilet paper and facial tissue when needed. Open the bathroom window for a short time, if possible, to air out the room. Once a week, wash out the waste can and laundry hamper. Launder the bath mats and rugs.

9. Store supplies.

10. Remove and discard gloves.

11. Wash your hands.

12. Document the cleaning.

Guidelines: Cleaning and Organizing Storage Areas

G Every item in the home should have a storage place that is convenient for use. That means storage places should be as close as possible to where they are used. For example, bath towels should be stored in or near the bathroom. Items that are used together should be stored near each other. Arrange food on shelves according to category. Store dangerous materials, such as cleaning products, out of reach of children and confused adults.

G Some storage areas only need to be cleaned occasionally. Remove the stored items. Wipe the shelves and drawers with a damp cloth and cleaner. Clean food storage areas more often.

G Do not change the client's or the family's storage arrangements without talking to them. If you think changes are needed, discuss your ideas with the family.

Most cleaning tasks should be done regularly, whether immediately, daily, weekly, monthly, or less often. The HHA will need to take into account the care plan, his assigned tasks, how much help is needed, and how much time he has in a particular home to prepare a cleaning schedule. He may not always follow the schedule exactly, but it will guide his work and help get essential cleaning done. Establishing a schedule can also help the family keep a housekeeping routine after home care has ended.

HHAs must follow Standard Precautions with every client. This is true because it is not possible to always know when infection is present. However, when a client has a known infectious disease, such as influenza, or one that weakens the immune system, such as AIDS or cancer, the HHA should take these special precautions in housecleaning:

- Use disinfectant when cleaning countertops and surfaces in the kitchen and bathroom.

- Clean the client's bathroom daily. Have other family members use a different bathroom if possible.

- Use separate dishes and utensils for the infected client.

- Wash dishes and utensils in the dishwasher or wash dishes in hot, soapy water with bleach. Rinse in boiling water, and allow to air dry.

- Disinfect any surfaces that come into contact with body fluids, such as bedpans, urinals, and toilets.

- Frequently remove trash containing used tissues.

- Keep any specimens of urine, stool, or sputum in double bags and away from food and food preparation areas.

Laundry

Hand or machine washing may be a part of an HHA's assignments. Clean clothes, bed linens, and towels are important for hygiene and comfort.

Laundry Products and Equipment: Washing laundry requires laundry detergent, a washing machine or a basin for hand-washing clothes, and a dryer or a clothesline and pins. The instructions for using washing machines are usually located on the inside of the machine lid. In general, it is best to use all-purpose detergent. High efficiency (HE) washing machines may require low-sudsing detergents that are compatible with these types of machines. Some delicate fabrics, underwear, or stockings may require a special detergent. Some clients may prefer a non-detergent soap for use on baby clothes and diapers. Bleach, color brighteners, stain removers, and fabric softeners may also be used. An HHA should ask the client and family about their preferences for laundry products.

Pretreating: Pretreating means giving special treatment to items that have heavy soil, spots, and stains before washing them. Spots and stains should be treated immediately. The sooner they are treated, the easier they are to remove. Some oily stains harden with age and cannot be removed. It helps to identify the source of the stain and treat it according to a stain guide on the pretreating solution.

Bleach: Bleach is used with detergent. However, bleach cannot be used on all fabrics. The HHA should be familiar with the type of bleach and the fabric that is being washed. Two types of bleach are used in laundry: chlorine bleach and non-chlorine (called *oxygen* or *all-fabric*) bleach. Each type of bleach should be used with caution. The instructions on the container should be read carefully.

Water Temperature: The HHA should read the washing instructions for all materials and garments. Warm water is the safest temperature for most garments. However, some must be washed in cold to prevent shrinking or colors from fading. Hot water is generally used for towels, bed linens, and white or colorfast cottons. Warm is usually used for permanent press, knit, synthetic, sheer, lace, acetate, fabric blends, and washable rayons. Cold water is used for brightly-colored fabrics or fabrics that are not colorfast.

Washing Action or Cycle: Cottons, linens, rayons, permanent press, knits, synthetics, blends, and most other items use the normal washer setting. The slow or gentle setting should be used for washable woolens, old quilts, curtains, and delicate or fragile items.

Drying Clothes: Settings on the dryer vary according to the model. The more delicate a fabric, the lower the drying temperature and the shorter the time in the dryer. Heavy items such as towels need higher temperature settings and a longer time in the dryer. The lint filter should be cleaned each time the dryer is used. If the client does not have a clothes dryer, the HHA can hang clothes on a clothesline using clothespins.

Folding: Removing all clothes from the dryer immediately will reduce wrinkling. Clothes can then be folded neatly or placed on hangers. If clothes need to be ironed, they may be set aside; other clothes should be put away in drawers or in a closet.

Ironing: Most care labels will indicate the best ironing temperature. If there is no tag, or no temperature is indicated, it is best to use the lowest temperature on the iron to avoid damaging the fabric. Pile fabrics like velvet and corduroy will keep their texture better if ironed on the wrong side over a towel. Dark fabrics, silks, acetates, rayons, linens, and some wools must be pressed on the wrong side to prevent them from becoming shiny. A pressing cloth can help protect the fabric.

Maintaining Clothing: An HHA may need to do basic mending or sewing occasionally. This is especially true if he is taking care of a family, an older person with impaired vision, or people who may not have the time or the ability to keep clothing and linens repaired. Some clients who can do their own mending may just need the HHA to thread the needle.

Doing the laundry

1. **Sort clothes carefully. Make separate piles of whites and colors. Check clothing labels for special washing instructions. Do not wash anything labeled** *Dry Clean Only*. **If hand washing is recommended, do not wash in the machine.**

2. **As you sort laundry, check pockets and remove tissues, money, pens, and other items. Remove belts with buckles, trims, and non-washable ornaments. Close zippers, buttons, and other fasteners. Check garments for stains and areas of heavy soil. If appropriate, mend or repair any holes, snags, rips, tears, pulled seams, and weak spots in garments and other items.**

3. **Pretreat spots and stains before washing (Fig. 6-1). A small amount of liquid detergent or dry detergent dissolved in water can be worked in with an old toothbrush. Pretreat or soak clothing as soon as possible for best results. If you know something is spotted, do not let it sit in the laundry hamper all week until you do the laundry.**

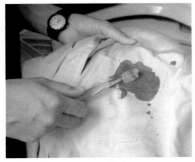

Fig. 6-1. Pretreating helps remove spots, stains, and areas that are heavily soiled.

4. **Use the correct water temperature: hot for whites, warm or cold for colors, cold for delicate fabrics.**

5. **Use the appropriate laundry product(s). Follow the washing instructions on the container.**

6. **Follow written instructions or client or family instructions for using the washer. Use the correct washing cycle for the load you are laundering.**

7. **Dry clothes completely, either in a dryer or on a clothesline. If using a dryer, follow the drying instructions on clothing labels or the client's preferences. Some fabrics require cooler temperatures.**

8. **Hand-wash items in warm or cool water, depending on the fabric and instructions. Use a mild detergent or special hand-washing liquid. Line dry or lay items flat on towels to preserve the shape of the garments.**

9. **Fold or hang clean laundry and sort into categories. Store in drawers or closets.**

When a client has a known infectious disease, the HHA must take these special precautions when handling laundry:

Guidelines: Handling Laundry for Infectious Clients

G   Keep client's laundry separate from other family members' laundry.

G   Handle dirty laundry as little as possible. Do not shake it. Sort it and put it in plastic bags in the client's room or bathroom. Take it immediately to the laundry area. Keep laundry off the floor.

G   Wear gloves and hold laundry away from your clothes and body when you are handling it.

G   Use liquid bleach when fabrics allow.

G   Use agency-approved disinfectants in all loads.

G   Use hot water.

In some assignments, an HHA will be asked to teach housekeeping skills to family members. This prepares them to take over housekeeping and care when home care is discontinued. By teaching household management skills, the HHA helps families meet their daily needs and become more self-reliant.

Guidelines: Teaching Family Members

G   Get to know the family before starting to teach them. Understand their needs or problems before beginning.

G   Be patient. Give people time to learn new skills. Praise their efforts.

G   Keep teaching sessions brief.

G   Break down tasks into simple steps. Explain each step and demonstrate it.

G   Answer all questions.

G   Assist the person as necessary. Do not do the task for him or her.

G   Remember that each person is an individual and will learn in different ways. Customize your teaching to allow for these differences.

Bedmaking

Some clients spend much or all of their time in bed. Careful bedmaking is essential for comfort, cleanliness, and health. Linens should always be changed after personal care, such as bed baths, or any time bedding or sheets are damp, soiled, or in need of straightening. Bed linens must be changed frequently for these reasons:

- Sheets that are damp, wrinkled, or bunched up are uncomfortable. They may prevent the client from resting or sleeping well.

- Microorganisms thrive in moist, warm environments. Bedding that is damp or unclean encourages infection and disease.

- Clients who spend long hours in bed are at risk for pressure ulcers. Sheets that do not lie flat under the client's body increase this risk by cutting off circulation.

Before handling clean linen, the HHA should wash her hands. Clean linen should not touch the HHA's uniform while she is carrying it. The HHA should don gloves before removing bed linen from the bed. When removing linen, she should fold or roll it so that the dirtiest area is inside.

If a client cannot get out of bed, an HHA must change the linens with the client in bed. An occupied bed is made while the client is in the bed. When making the bed, the HHA should use a wide stance and bend her knees. Bending from the waist should be avoided, especially when tucking sheets under the mattress. Mattresses can be heavy. It is easier to make an empty bed than one with a client in it. An unoccupied bed is a bed made while no client is in the bed. If the client can be moved, the HHA's job will be easier.

Making an occupied bed

Equipment: clean linen—mattress pad, fitted or flat bottom sheet, waterproof bed protector (if needed), cotton draw sheet, flat top sheet, blanket(s), bath blanket, pillowcase(s), gloves

1. Wash your hands.

2. Explain the procedure to the client, speaking clearly, slowly, and directly. Maintain face-to-face contact whenever possible.

3. Provide privacy if the client desires it.

4. Place clean linen on clean surface within reach (e.g., bedside stand or chair).

5. If the bed is adjustable, adjust bed to a safe level, usually waist high. Lower the head of the bed. If the bed is movable, lock bed wheels.

6. Put on gloves.

7. Loosen top linen from the end of the bed on the working side.

8. Unfold the bath blanket over the top sheet to cover the client, and remove the top sheet. Keep the client covered at all times with the bath blanket.

9. You will make the bed one side at a time. Raise side rail (if bed has them) on far side of bed. This prevents the client from falling out of the bed while you are making it. After raising the side rail, go to the other side of bed. Help client to turn onto her side, moving away from you, toward the raised side rail.

10. Loosen the bottom soiled linen, mattress pad, and protector, if present, on the working side.

11. Roll bottom soiled linen toward client, soiled side inside. Tuck it snugly against the client's back.

12. Place and tuck in clean bottom linen, finishing with bottom sheet free of wrinkles. If you are using a flat bottom sheet, leave enough overlap on each end to tuck under the mattress. If the sheet is only long enough to tuck in at one end, tuck it in securely at the top of the bed. Make hospital corners to keep bottom sheet wrinkle-free (Fig. 6-2).

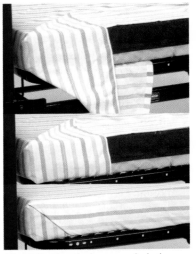

Fig. 6-2. Hospital corners help keep the flat sheet smooth under the client. They help prevent a client's feet from being restricted by or tangled in linen when getting in and out of bed.

13. Smooth the bottom sheet out toward the client. Be sure there are no wrinkles in the mattress pad. Roll the extra material toward the client and tuck it under the client's body.

14. If using a waterproof bed protector, unfold it and center it on

the bed. Tuck the side near you under the mattress. Smooth it out toward the client, and tuck as you did with the sheet.

15. If using a draw sheet, place it on the bed. Tuck in on your side, smooth, and tuck as you did with the other bedding.

16. Raise side rail nearest you. Go to the other side of the bed and lower the side rail on that side. Help client turn onto clean bottom sheet. Protect the client from any soiled matter on the old linens.

17. Loosen the soiled linen. Check for any personal items. Roll linen from head to the foot of the bed. Avoid contact with your skin or clothes. Place it in a hamper or basket. Never put it on the floor or furniture. Never shake it. Soiled bed linens are full of microorganisms that should not be spread to other parts of the room.

18. Pull the clean linen through as quickly as possible. Start with the mattress pad and wrap around corners. Pull and tuck in clean bottom linen just like the other side. Pull and tuck in waterproof bed protector and draw sheet if used. Finish with bottom sheet free of wrinkles.

19. Ask client to turn onto her back. Help as needed. Keep client covered and comfortable, with a pillow under her head. Raise the side rail.

20. Unfold the top sheet. Place it over the client and center it. Ask the client to hold the top sheet. Slip the bath blanket or old sheet out from underneath. Put it in the laundry hamper.

21. Place a blanket over the top sheet, matching the top edges.

Tuck the bottom edges of top sheet and blanket under the bottom of the mattress. Make hospital corners on each side. Loosen the top linens over the client's feet. This prevents pressure on the feet. At the top of the bed, fold the top sheet over the blanket about six inches.

22. Remove the pillow. Do not hold it near your face. Remove the soiled pillowcase by turning it inside out. Place it in the laundry hamper.

23. Remove and discard gloves. Wash your hands.

24. With one hand, grasp the clean pillowcase at the closed end. Turn it inside out over your arm. Next, using the same hand that has the pillowcase over it, grasp one narrow edge of the pillow. Pull the pillowcase over it with your free hand (Fig. 6-3). Do the same for any other pillows. Place them under your client's head with open end away from the door, or as client desires.

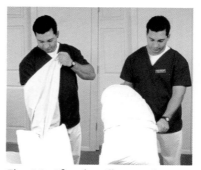

Fig. 6-3. *After the pillowcase is turned inside out over your arm, grasp one end of the pillow. Pull the pillowcase over the pillow.*

25. If you raised an adjustable bed, return it to its lowest position.

Leave side rails in the ordered position. Put any signaling device within the client's reach. Carry laundry hamper to laundry area.

26. Wash your hands.

27. Document the procedure and any observations.

Making an unoccupied bed

Equipment: clean linen—mattress pad, fitted or flat bottom sheet, waterproof bed protector (if needed), cotton draw sheet, flat top sheet, blanket(s), pillowcase(s), gloves

1. Wash your hands.

2. Place clean linen on clean surface within reach (e.g., bedside stand or chair).

3. If the bed is adjustable, adjust bed to a safe level, usually waist high. Put bed in flattest position. If the bed is movable, lock bed wheels.

4. Put on gloves.

5. Loosen soiled linen. Roll soiled linen (soiled side inside) from head to foot of bed. Avoid contact with your skin or clothes. Place it in a hamper or basket. Do not put it on the floor or furniture. Remove pillows and pillowcases and place pillowcases in hamper.

6. Remove and discard gloves. Wash your hands.

7. Remake the bed. Start with the mattress pad and wrap around corners. Place bottom sheet, tucking under mattress. Make hospital corners to keep bottom sheet wrinkle-free. Put on waterproof bed protector and draw sheet, if used, smooth, and tuck under sides of bed.

8. Place top sheet and blanket over bed. Center these, tuck under end of bed, and make hospital corners. Fold down the top sheet over the blanket about six inches. Fold both top sheet and blanket down so client can easily get into bed. If client will not be returning to bed immediately, leave bedding up.

9. Put on clean pillowcases (as described in procedure on previous page). Replace pillows.

10. If you raised an adjustable bed, return it to its lowest position.

11. Carry laundry hamper to laundry area.

12. Wash your hands.

13. Document the procedure and any observations.

Proper Nutrition

Nutrition

Proper nutrition is very important. Nutrition is how the body uses food to maintain health. Bodies need a well-balanced diet with nutrients and plenty of fluids. This helps the body grow new cells, maintain normal body function, and have energy. Proper nutrition in early life helps ensure good health later in life. For the ill or elderly, a well-balanced diet helps maintain muscle and skin tissue and prevent pressure ulcers. A healthy diet promotes healing. It also helps a person cope with stress.

A nutrient is a substance that is necessary for growth and life. Nutrients provide energy, promote growth and health, and help regulate metabolism. Metabolism is the process by which nutrients are broken down to be used by the body for energy and other needs. The body needs the following six nutrients for growth and development:

1. **Water**: Water is the most essential nutrient for life. One-half to two-thirds of the body's weight is water. A person needs about 64 ounces, or eight 8-ounce glasses, of water or other fluids per day. Without it, a person can only live a few days. Water assists in the digestion and absorption of food. It helps with waste elimination. Through perspiration, water also helps maintain normal body temperature. Maintaining fluid balance in the body is necessary for good health. The fluids a person drinks—water, juice, soda, coffee, tea, and milk—provide most of the water the body uses. Some foods are also sources of water, including soup, celery, lettuce, apples, and peaches.

2. **Carbohydrates**: Carbohydrates supply the body with energy and extra protein. They help the body use fat efficiently. Carbohydrates also provide fiber, which is necessary for bowel elimination. Carbohydrates can be divided into two basic types: complex and simple carbohydrates. Complex carbohydrates are found in bread, cereal, potatoes, rice, pasta, vegetables, and fruits. Simple carbohydrates are found in sugars, sweets, syrups, and jellies. Simple carbohydrates do not have the same nutritional value that complex carbohydrates do.

3. **Protein**: Proteins are part of every body cell. They are essential for tissue growth and repair. Proteins also supply energy for the body. Excess proteins are excreted by the kidneys or stored as body fat. Sources of protein include seafood, poultry, meat, eggs, milk, cheese, nuts, nut butters, peas, beans or legumes, and soy products (tofu, tempeh, some veggie burgers). Whole grain cereals, pastas, rice, and breads contain some proteins, too.

4. **Fats**: Fat helps the body store energy. In addition, fats add flavor to food. Fats also help the body absorb certain vitamins. Excess fat in the diet is stored as fat in the body. Examples of fats are butter, margarine, salad dressings, oils, and animal fats found in meats, dairy products, fowl, and fish. Monounsaturated vegetable fats (including olive oil and canola oil) and polyunsaturated vegetable fats (including corn and safflower oils) are healthier fats. Saturated fats, including animal fats like butter, lard, bacon, and other fatty meats, are not as healthy. They should be limited.

5. **Vitamins**: Vitamins are substances needed by the body to function. The body cannot produce most vitamins. They can only be obtained from certain foods. Vitamins A, D, E, and K are fat-soluble vitamins. This means they are carried and stored in body fat. Vitamins B and C are water-soluble vitamins. They are broken down by water in the body and used by the body, but cannot be stored. Excess B and C vitamins are eliminated in urine and feces.

6. **Minerals**: Minerals maintain body functions. Minerals help build bones, make hormones, and help in blood formation. They provide energy and control body processes. Zinc, iron, calcium, and magnesium are examples of minerals. Minerals are found in many foods.

Most foods contain several nutrients, but no one food has all the nutrients needed for a healthy body. This is why it is important to eat a daily diet that is well-balanced. There is not one single dietary plan that is right for everyone. People have different nutritional needs, depending upon their age, gender, and activity level.

In 2011, the U.S. Department of Agriculture (USDA) developed MyPlate to help people build a healthy plate at meal times (Fig. 6-4). The MyPlate icon emphasizes vegetables, fruits, grains, protein, and low-fat dairy products.

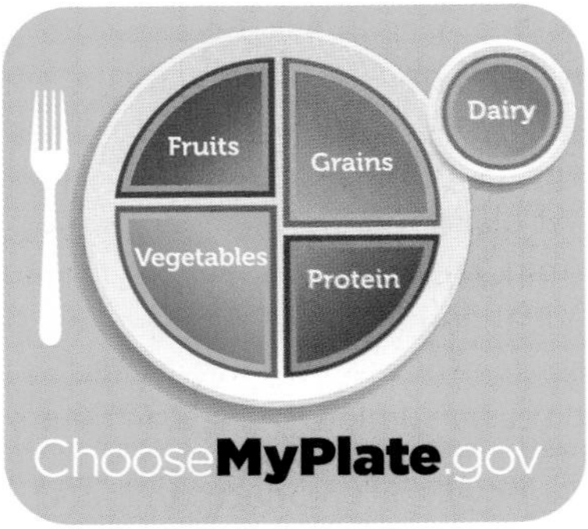

MyPlate gives suggestions and tools for making healthy choices. It does not provide specific messages about what a person should eat. The My Plate icon includes the following food groups:

Fig. 6-4. The U.S. Department of Agriculture developed the MyPlate icon (ChooseMyPlate.gov) to help promote healthy eating practices.

Vegetables and fruits: A person should make half his plate fruits and vegetables. Vegetables include all fresh, frozen, canned, and dried vegetables, and vegetable juices. There are five subgroups within the vegetable group, organized by their nutritional content. These are dark green vegetables, red and orange vegetables, dry beans and peas, starchy vegetables, and other vegetables. A variety of vegetables from these subgroups should be eaten every day. Dark green, red, and orange vegetables have the best nutritional content.

Fruits include all fresh, frozen, canned, and dried fruits, and 100% fruit juices. Most choices should be whole, cut-up, or pureed fruit, rather than juice, for the additional dietary fiber provided. Fruit can be added as a main dish, side dish, or as a dessert.

Grains: A person should make half his grain intake whole grains. There are many different grains. Some common ones are wheat, rice, oats, corn, and barley. Foods made from grains include bread, pasta, oatmeal, breakfast cereals, tortillas, and grits. Grains can be divided into two groups: whole grains and refined grains. Whole grains contain bran and germ, as well as the endosperm. Refined grains retain only the endosperm. The endosperm is the tissue within flowering plants. It surrounds and nourishes the plant embryo. Examples of whole grains include brown rice, wild rice, bulgur, whole-grain corn, whole oats, whole wheat, and whole rye. Foods rich in fiber reduce the risk of heart disease and other diseases and may reduce constipation.

Protein: MyPlate guidelines emphasize the importance of eating a variety of protein foods every week. Meat, poultry, seafood, and eggs are animal sources of proteins. Beans, peas, soy products, nuts, and seeds are plant sources of proteins. Seafood should be eaten twice a week in place of meat or poultry. Seafood that is higher in oils and low in mercury, such as salmon or trout, is a good choice. Lean meats and poultry, as well as eggs and egg whites, can be eaten on a regular basis. A person should eat plant-based protein foods more often. Beans and peas, soy products (tofu, tempeh, some veggie burgers), nuts, and seeds are low in saturated fat and high in fiber. Some nuts and seeds (flax, walnuts) are excellent sources of essential fatty acids. These acids may reduce the risk of heart disease. Sunflower seeds and almonds are good sources of vitamin E.

Dairy: All milk products and foods made from milk that retain their calcium content, such as yogurt and cheese, are part of the dairy category. Most dairy group choices should be fat-free or low-fat (1%). Fat-free or low-fat milk or yogurt should be chosen more often than cheese. Milk and yogurt contain less sodium than most cheeses. Milk provides nutrients that are vital for the health and maintenance of the body. These nutrients include calcium, potassium, vitamin D, and protein. Fat-free or low-fat milk provides these nutrients without the extra calories and saturated fat. Soy products enriched with calcium are an alternative to dairy foods.

Most clients should be encouraged to drink at least 64 ounces of water or other fluids a day. Water is an essential nutrient for life. The sense of thirst can lessen as people age. Infection, fever, diarrhea, and some medications will also increase the need for fluid intake. HHAs should remind elderly clients to drink fluids often. Some clients will drink more fluids if they are offered to them in smaller amounts, rather than one large glassful. However, some clients may have an order to restrict fluids (RF) or to force fluids (FF) because of medical conditions. The abbreviation *NPO* stands for *nothing by mouth*. This means that a client is not allowed to have anything to eat or to drink, not even water. The HHA should follow each client's care plan.

Dehydration occurs when a person does not have enough fluid in the body. Dehydration is a serious condition. People can become dehydrated if they do not drink enough or if they have diarrhea or are vomiting. Preventing dehydration is very important.

Guidelines: Preventing Dehydration

G   Report observations and warning signs to your supervisor immediately.

G   Encourage clients to drink every time you see them.

G   Offer fresh water or other fluids often. Offer drinks that the client enjoys. Some may not like water and may prefer other types of beverages, such as juice, soda, tea, or milk. Some clients do not want ice in their drinks. Honor personal preferences.

G   Ice chips, frozen flavored ice sticks, and gelatin are also forms of liquids. Offer them often. Do not offer ice chips or sticks if a client has a swallowing problem.

G   If appropriate, offer sips of liquid between bites of food at meals and during snack time.

G   Make sure a pitcher and cup are near enough and light enough for a client to lift.

G   Offer assistance if a client cannot drink without help. Use adaptive cups as needed.

G   Record fluid intake and output if assigned.

Observing and Reporting: Dehydration

O/R   Client drinks less than eight 8-ounce glasses of liquid per day

O/R   Client drinks little or no fluids at meals

O/R   Client needs help drinking from a cup or glass

O/R   Client has trouble swallowing liquids

O/R   Client has frequent vomiting, diarrhea, or fever

O/R   Client is easily tired or confused

In addition, report any of these symptoms:

- %R Dry mouth
- %R Cracked lips
- %R Sunken eyes
- %R Dark urine
- %R Strong-smelling urine
- %R Weight loss
- %R Complaints of abdominal pain

Fluid overload occurs when the body cannot handle the amount of fluid consumed. This condition often affects people with heart or kidney disease.

Observing and Reporting: Fluid Overload

- %R Swelling/edema of extremities (ankles, feet, fingers, hands)
- %R Weight gain (daily weight gain of one to two pounds)
- %R Decreased urine output
- %R Shortness of breath
- %R Increased heart rate
- %R Anxiety
- %R Skin that appears tight, smooth, and shiny

Aging and illness can lead to emotional and physical problems that affect the intake of food. For example, people who are lonely or who suffer from illnesses that affect their ability to chew and swallow may have little interest in food. Unintended weight loss is a serious problem for the elderly. Weight loss can mean that the client has a serious medical condition. It can lead to skin breakdown, which leads to pressure ulcers. It is very important for HHAs to report any weight loss, no matter how small.

Guidelines: Preventing Unintended Weight Loss

- G Report observations and warning signs to your supervisor.
- G Food should look, taste, and smell good. The client may have a poor sense of taste and smell.
- G Encourage clients to eat. Talk about food being served in a positive tone of voice. Use positive words.
- G Honor clients' food likes and dislikes.
- G Offer different kinds of foods and beverages.

G   Help clients who have trouble feeding themselves.

G   Season foods to clients' preferences, following dietary orders.

G   Allow time for clients to finish eating.

G   Notify your supervisor if clients have trouble using utensils.

G   Record the meal/snack intake if assigned.

G   Provide oral care before or after meals and as the client requests it.

G   Position clients sitting upright for eating.

G   If a client has had a loss of appetite and/or seems sad, ask about it.

Observing and Reporting: Unintended Weight Loss

O/R   Client needs help eating or drinking

O/R   Client eats less than 70% of meals/snacks served

O/R   Client has mouth pain

O/R   Client has dentures that do not fit properly

O/R   Client has difficulty chewing or swallowing (dysphagia)

O/R   Client coughs or chokes while eating

O/R   Client is sad, has crying spells, or withdraws from others

O/R   Client is confused, wanders, or paces

Clients with swallowing problems may be restricted to consuming only thickened liquids. Thickened liquids have a thickening powder or agent added to them. This improves the ability to control fluid in the mouth and throat. A doctor orders the necessary thickness after the client has been evaluated by a speech-language pathologist. If thickening is ordered, it must be used with all liquids. This means that HHAs should not offer regular liquids, such as water or other beverages, to a client who must have thickened liquids. There are three basic thickened consistencies:

1. **Nectar Thick**: This consistency is thicker than water. It is the thickness of a thick juice, such as pear nectar or tomato juice. A client can drink this from a cup.

2. **Honey Thick**: This consistency has the thickness of honey. It will pour very slowly. A client will usually use a spoon to consume it.

3. **Pudding Thick**: With this consistency, the liquids have become semi-solid, much like pudding. A spoon should stand up straight in the glass when put into the middle of the drink. A client must consume these liquids with a spoon.

Swallowing problems put clients at high risk for choking on food or drink. Inhaling food, fluid, or foreign material into the lungs is called **aspiration**. Aspiration can cause pneumonia or death. An HHA should notify the supervisor immediately if any problems occur while feeding.

Guidelines: Preventing Aspiration

G   Position clients in a straight, upright position when eating or drinking. Do not try to feed clients in a reclining position.

G   Offer small pieces of food or small spoonfuls of pureed food.

G   Feed clients slowly. Do not rush them.

G   Place food in the unaffected, or stronger, side of the mouth.

G   Make sure mouth is empty before each bite of food or sip of drink.

G   Keep clients in the upright position for at least 30 minutes after eating and drinking.

When the digestive system does not function properly, hyperalimentation or total parenteral nutrition (TPN) may be needed. With TPN, a solution of nutrients goes directly into the bloodstream. It bypasses the digestive system.

When a person is unable to swallow, he or she may be fed through a tube. A nasogastric tube is inserted into the nose and goes to the stomach. A tube can also be placed into the stomach through the abdominal wall. This is called a *percutaneous endoscopic gastrostomy (PEG) tube*. The surgically-created opening into the stomach that allows the insertion of a tube is called a *gastrostomy* (Fig. 6-5). Tube feedings are used when clients cannot swallow but can digest food.

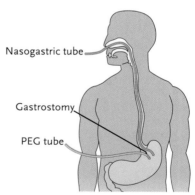

Fig. 6-5. *Nasogastric tubes are inserted through the nose. PEG tubes are inserted through the abdominal wall into the stomach.*

Home health aides are not responsible for tube feedings. HHAs do not insert or remove tubes, do the feeding, or irrigate (clean) the tubes. They may assemble equipment and supplies. HHAs may position the client in a sitting position for feeding, and they may also discard or clean and store used equipment and supplies. In addition, HHAs may observe, report, and document any changes in the client or problems with the feeding.

When planning meals and cooking for clients, HHAs need to know their food preferences. Some of these may be listed in the care plan. The HHA should ask the client or a family member to tell her about food preferences, or suggest some sample menus and ask for reactions. She should pay attention to what is eaten when she serves meals. If a client never finishes his chicken, it may mean that he prefers other kinds of meats. Cost may also be a factor in choosing foods. Protein-rich foods are generally the most expensive, but also the most important for the healing process.

The Food and Drug Administration (FDA) (fda.gov) requires that all packaged foods contain a standardized nutrition label, called *Nutrition Facts*. The Nutrition Facts label gives the following information:

- Serving size and number of servings per container
- Calories per serving
- Percentage of the recommended daily values a serving contains
- Amount of added sugars
- Percentage of recommended daily totals for certain vitamins and minerals

Special Diets

A doctor sometimes places clients who are ill on special diets. These diets are known as *therapeutic, modified,* or *special diets*. Certain nutrients or fluids may need to be restricted or removed. Some medications may interact with certain foods, which then must be eliminated. Doctors may order special diets for clients who do not eat enough. Diets are also prescribed for weight control and food allergies.

The care plan should specify any special diet the client is on. Therapeutic diets can only be prescribed by doctors and planned by dietitians. An HHA must never modify a client's diet and should follow the client's diet plan.

Low-Sodium Diet: Clients with high blood pressure, heart disease, kidney disease, or fluid retention may be placed on a low-sodium diet. Many foods have sodium, but people are most familiar with it as an ingredient in table salt. Salt is the first food to be restricted in a low-sodium diet because it is high in sodium. Clients on a low-sodium diet should avoid high-sodium foods and adding salt to foods. Foods high in sodium include cured meats, such as ham, bacon, lunch meat, sausage, salt pork, and hot dogs; salty or smoked fish, including herring, salted cod, sardines, anchovies, caviar, smoked salmon, or lox; processed cheese and some other cheeses; salted foods, including nuts, pretzels, potato chips, dips, and spreads; vegetables preserved in brine, such as pickles, sauerkraut, pickled vegetables, olives, and relishes; sauces with high concentrations of salt, including Worcestershire, barbecue, chili, steak, and soy sauces; ketchup, mustard, and mayonnaise; commercially-prepared foods, such as breads, canned soups and vegetables, and certain breakfast cereals; and gelatin dessert. Some over-the-counter medications are also high in sodium.

For clients on a low-sodium diet, product labels should be read to determine if they contain salt or sodium in any form. Low-sodium meals can be made more flavorful by adding lemon, herbs, dry mustard, pepper, paprika, orange rind, onion, and garlic to recipes. The flavor of meats can also be enhanced by the addition of fruits and jellies.

Common abbreviations for this diet are *Low Na*, which means low sodium, or *NAS*, which stands for *No Added Salt*.

Fluid-Restricted Diet: The fluid taken into the body through food and fluids must equal the amount of fluid that leaves the body through perspiration, stool, urine, and expiration. This is fluid balance. When fluid intake is greater than fluid output, body tissues become swollen with fluid. People with severe heart disease and kidney disease may have trouble processing fluid. To prevent further damage, doctors may restrict fluid intake. For clients on fluid restriction, the HHA will measure and document exact amounts of fluid intake and report excesses to the supervisor. Additional fluids or foods that count as fluids, such as ice cream, puddings, gelatin, etc., should not be offered. If the client complains of thirst or requests fluids, the HHA should tell her supervisor. A common abbreviation for this diet is *RF*, which stands for *Restrict Fluids*.

High-Potassium Diet (K+): Some clients are taking blood pressure medications or diuretics, which are medications that reduce fluid volume. These clients may be excreting so much fluid that their bodies are depleted of potassium. Other clients may be placed on a high-potassium diet for different reasons.

Foods high in potassium include bananas, grapefruit, oranges, orange juice, prune juice, prunes, dried apricots, figs, raisins, dates, cantaloupes, tomatoes, potatoes with skins, sweet potatoes and yams, winter squash, legumes, avocados, and unsalted nuts. *K+* is the common abbreviation for this diet.

Low-Protein Diet: People who have kidney disease may also be on low-protein diets. Protein is restricted because it breaks down into compounds that may lead to further kidney damage. The extent of the restriction depends on the stage of the disease and if the client is on dialysis. Vegetables and starches, such as breads and pasta, are encouraged.

Low-Fat/Low-Cholesterol Diet: People who have high levels of cholesterol in their blood are at risk for heart attacks and heart disease. People with gallbladder disease, diseases that interfere with fat digestion, and liver disease are also placed on low-fat/low-cholesterol diets. This diet permits skim milk, low-fat cottage cheese, fish, white meat of turkey and chicken, fresh fruits and vegetables, and vegetable fats (especially monounsaturated fats such as olive and canola oils). Clients on this diet may need to follow these guidelines:

- Eat lean cuts of meat, including lamb, beef, and pork, and eat these only three times a week.
- Limit egg yolks to three or four per week (including eggs used in baking).
- Avoid organ meats, shellfish, fatty meats, cream, butter, lard, meat drippings, coconut and palm oils, and desserts and soups made with whole milk.
- Avoid fried foods and sweets.

People who have gallbladder disease or other digestive problems may be placed on a diet that restricts all fats. A common abbreviation for this diet is *Low-Fat/Low-Chol*.

Modified Calorie Diet: Some clients may need to reduce calories to lose weight or prevent weight gain. Other clients need to increase calories because of malnutrition, surgery, illness, or fever. Common abbreviations for this diet are *Low-Cal* or *High-Cal*.

Bland Diet: Gastric and duodenal ulcers can be irritated by foods that produce or increase levels of acid in the stomach, so these foods are eliminated. The bland diet is also used for people who have intestinal disorders, such as Crohn's disease or irritable bowel syndrome (IBS). The following foods and drinks should be avoided: alcohol; beverages containing caffeine, such as coffee, tea, and soft drinks; citrus juices; spicy foods; and spicy seasonings such as black pepper, cayenne, and chili pepper. Three meals or more a day are usually advised. If alcohol is allowed, it should be drunk with meals.

Diabetic Diet: Calories and carbohydrates are carefully controlled in the diets of clients who have diabetes. Protein and fats are also regulated. The foods and the amounts are determined by nutritional and energy needs. A dietitian and the client will make up a meal plan. It will include all the right types and amounts of food for each day. The meal plan may use a carbohydrate-counting approach (often called *carb counting*). After the proper amount of carbohydrates is determined by the dietitian, they need to be counted in each meal or snack. Meal planning can also be done by using the exchange system. In this system, similar foods can be substituted for one another to make up a menu. Looking at the exchange list, the client makes food choices while controlling his diet.

To keep their blood glucose levels near normal, diabetic clients must eat the right amount of the right type of food at the right time. They must eat all that is served. HHAs should encourage them to do so. HHAs should not offer other foods without the doctor's approval. If a client will not eat what is directed, or is not following the diet, the HHA should inform the supervisor.

Diabetics should avoid foods that are high in sugar because sugary foods can cause problems with insulin balance. Foods and drinks high in sugar include candy, ice cream, cakes, cookies, jellies, jams, fruits canned in heavy syrup, soft drinks, and alcoholic beverages. Many foods are high in sugar that do not appear to be so, such as canned fruits and vegetables, many breakfast cereals, and ketchup. The American Diabetes Association's (ADA) website, diabetes.org, has more information.

Low-Residue (Low-Fiber) Diet: This diet decreases the amount of fiber, whole grains, raw fruits and vegetables, seeds, and other foods, such as dairy and coffee. The low-residue diet is used for people with bowel disturbances.

High-Residue (High-Fiber) Diet: High-residue diets increase the intake of fiber and whole grains, such as whole grain cereals, bread, and raw fruits and vegetables. This diet helps with problems such as constipation and bowel disorders.

Gluten-Free Diet: This diet is free of gluten, which is a protein found in wheat, rye, and barley. It is used for people with celiac disease, which is a disorder that can damage the intestines if gluten is consumed. Foods containing wheat flour, such as tortillas, crackers, breads, cakes, pastas, and cereals, are eliminated from the diet. Some sauces and dressings also have wheat in them. Other items that may contain gluten include beer, hot dogs, candy, broths, and medications.

Unlike celiac disease, gluten intolerance is a condition that does not cause damage to the intestines. It does, however, cause unpleasant symptoms such as abdominal pain, gas, and diarrhea when products containing gluten are consumed. If a person has a gluten intolerance, eliminating gluten from the diet is usually enough to manage symptoms.

Vegetarian Diet: Health issues may cause a person to require a vegetarian diet. A person may also choose to eat a vegetarian diet for religious reasons, or due to a dislike of meat, a compassion for animals, a belief in non-violence, or financial issues. Different types of vegetarian diets are

- A lacto-ovo vegetarian diet excludes all meats, fish, and poultry, but allows eggs and dairy products.
- A lacto-vegetarian diet eliminates poultry, meats, fish, and eggs, but allows dairy products.
- An ovo-vegetarian diet omits all meats, fish, poultry, and dairy products, but allows eggs.
- A vegan diet eliminates poultry, meats, fish, eggs, and dairy products, along with all foods that are derived from animals.

Diets may also be modified in consistency:

Liquid Diet: A liquid diet is usually ordered for a short time due to a medical condition or before or after a test or surgery. It is ordered when a client needs to keep the intestinal tract free of food. A liquid diet consists of foods that are in a liquid state at body temperature. Liquid diets are usually ordered as *clear* or *full*. A clear liquid diet includes clear juices, broth, gelatin, and popsicles. A full liquid diet includes all the liquids served on a clear liquid diet, with the addition of cream soups, milk, and ice cream.

Soft Diet and Mechanical Soft Diet: The soft diet is soft in texture and consists of soft or chopped foods that are easier to chew and swallow. Foods that are hard to chew and swallow, such as raw fruits and vegetables and some meats, will be restricted. High-fiber foods, fried foods, and spicy foods may also be limited. Doctors order this diet for clients who have trouble chewing and swallowing due to dental problems or other medical conditions. It is also ordered for people who are making the transition from a liquid diet to a regular diet.

The mechanical soft diet consists of chopped or blended foods that are easier to chew and swallow. Foods are prepared with blenders, food processors, meat grinders, or cutting utensils. Unlike the soft diet, the mechanical soft diet does not limit spices, fat, and fiber. Only the texture of foods is changed. For example, meats and poultry can be ground and moistened with sauces or water to ease swallowing. This diet is used for people recovering from surgery or who have difficulty chewing and swallowing.

Pureed Diet: To puree a food means to blend or grind it into a thick paste of baby food consistency. The food should be thick enough to hold its form in the mouth. This diet does not require a person to chew his food.

A pureed diet is often used for people who have trouble chewing and/or swallowing more textured foods.

Planning and Shopping

Home health aides should plan meals for a week or at least several days before shopping. When the meal plan is complete, the HHA can make a shopping list. On a large sheet of paper, she can list categories, including produce, meats, canned goods, frozen foods, dairy, and other. She should leave space under each category to list the foods she needs to buy. Listing items by category saves time in the grocery store. The HHA can go through the plan meal by meal and write down all of the ingredients needed for each meal. Beverages should be included as well. The HHA should check the refrigerator, cabinets, and pantry for ingredients. Many ingredients may already be in the home. It is a good idea to keep a shopping list available so family members, clients, and the HHA can write down things they run out of during the week.

Guidelines: Shopping for Clients

G   Use coupons. If your client receives a newspaper, scan it for coupons from stores or manufacturers. Coupons might also be available online or through a smartphone app. Use only those coupons for items you have already planned to buy.

G   Check websites, apps, or store circulars for advertised specials.

G   Buy fresh foods that are in season, when they are at peak flavor and inexpensive.

G   Buy in quantity. Large amounts or larger sizes are usually more economical, but do not buy more than the client can store.

G   Shop from your list. Do not be tempted by items that are not on your list.

G   Avoid processed, already-mixed, or ready-made foods. They are usually more expensive and less nutritious. When time allows, buy staples, or basic items.

G   Loaves of bread are generally a better buy than rolls or crackers. Day-old bread is usually sold at reduced prices.

G   Milk can be bought in many forms. Choose the type that the client prefers. Skim, one percent, or two percent milk contains lower fat and is usually cheaper than whole milk.

G   Buy a cheaper brand when appearance is not important.

G   Read labels to be sure you are getting the kind of product and the quantity you want.

G   Estimate the cost per serving before buying. Divide the total cost by the number of servings to determine the cost per serving.

G   Consider the amount of waste in bones and fat when buying cheaper cuts of meat.

G   Avoid convenience stores. Shopping at large supermarkets or discount stores usually guarantees the best prices.

G   Plan ahead. Knowing what a client needs before it runs out will save money.

When deciding what to buy, an HHA should keep these four factors in mind:

1. Nutritional value

2. Quality

3. Price

4. Preference

Preparing and Storing

Foodborne illnesses affect up to 100 million people each year. Elderly people are at increased risk partly because they may not see, smell, or taste that food is spoiled. They also may not have the energy to prepare and store food safely. For people who have weakened immune systems because of AIDS or cancer, a foodborne illness can be deadly.

Guidelines: Safe Food Preparation

G   Wash hands frequently. Wash your hands thoroughly before beginning any food preparation. Wash your hands after touching non-food items, and after handling raw meat, poultry, or fish.

G   Keep your hair tied back or covered. Wear clean clothes or a clean apron.

G   Wear gloves when you have a cut or wound on your hands.

G   Avoid coughing or sneezing around food. If you cough or sneeze, wash your hands immediately.

G   Keep everything clean. Clean and disinfect countertops and other surfaces before, during (as necessary), and after food preparation.

G   Handle raw meat, poultry, and fish carefully. Use an antibacterial kitchen cleaner or a dilute bleach solution to clean any countertops on which meat juices were spilled. Wrap paper or packaging containing meat juices in plastic and discard immediately.

G Once you have used a knife or cutting board to cut fresh meat, do not use it for anything else until it has been washed in hot, soapy water, rinsed in clear water, and allowed to air dry.

G Use one cutting board for fresh produce and bread, and a separate cutting board for raw meat, poultry, and seafood.

G Use hot, soapy water to wash utensils.

G Use clean dishcloths, sponges, and towels. Change them frequently. Sponges may be washed in the dishwasher to disinfect them.

G Defrost frozen foods in the refrigerator, not on the countertop. Do not remove meats or dairy products from the refrigerator until just before use.

G Wash fruits and vegetables thoroughly in running water to remove pesticides and bacteria.

G Cook meats, poultry, and fish thoroughly to kill any harmful micro-organisms they may contain. Heat leftovers thoroughly. Never leave food out for over two hours. Keep cold foods cold and hot foods hot.

G Do not use cracked eggs. Do not consume or serve raw eggs.

G Never taste and stir with the same utensil.

Cooking Safety

- Never work wearing loose or flowing clothing, especially around the stove. Roll up clients' sleeves and avoid loose clothing when client may be cooking or around the stove.
- Turn pot handles toward the back of the stove to prevent tipping.
- Dry hands before using electrical appliances.
- Immediately clean any spills on the floor to prevent slipping.
- Store potholders, dish towels, and other flammable items away from the stove.
- Stay in or near the kitchen when anything is cooking or baking. Never leave stove on and unattended.

The following basic methods of food preparation will allow the HHA to prepare a variety of healthy meals:

Boiling: Food is cooked in boiling water until tender or done. This is the best method for cooking pasta, noodles, rice, and hard- or soft-boiled eggs.

Steaming: Steaming is a healthy way to prepare vegetables. A small amount of water is boiled in the bottom of a saucepan and food is set over it on a rack or colander. The pan is tightly covered to keep the steam in (Fig. 6-6).

Poaching: Fish or eggs may be cooked by poaching in barely boiling water or other liquids. Eggs are cracked and shells discarded before poaching. Fish may be poached in broth, wine, milk, or other liquids on top of the stove or in the oven in a baking dish.

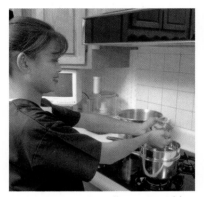

Fig. 6-6. *Steaming allows vegetables to retain their vitamins and flavor.*

Roasting: Used for meats and poultry or some vegetables, roasting is a simple way to cook. Dry heat roasting means food is roasted in an open pan in the oven. Meats and poultry are basted, or coated with juices or other liquid, during roasting.

Braising: Braising is a slow-cooking method that uses moist heat. Liquid such as broth, wine, or sauce is poured over and around meat or vegetables, and the pot is covered. The meat or vegetables are then slowly cooked at a temperature just below boiling. Braising is a good way to tenderize tough meats and vegetables, since the long cooking breaks down their fibers. Braising may be done in the oven or on the stove top.

Baking: Baking is used for many foods, including breads, poultry, fish, and vegetables. Baking is done at a moderate heat, 350°F to 400°F. Foods such as potatoes and winter squash bake very well.

Broiling: Used primarily for meats, broiling involves cooking food close to the source of heat at a high temperature for a short time. Meat must be tender to be broiled successfully. Inexpensive and lean cuts are often better cooked using moist heat. The *broil* setting on the oven can also be used to melt cheese or brown the top of a casserole. An HHA should leave the oven door ajar and never leave the kitchen when broiling; things can burn very fast.

Sautéing or stir-frying: These are quick cooking methods for vegetables and meats. Use a small amount of oil in a frying pan or wok over high heat.

Microwaving: Microwave ovens are used for defrosting, reheating, and cooking. However, cold spots can occur in microwaved foods. To minimize cold spots, food should be stirred and rotated once or twice during cooking. Food should be placed in microwave-safe bowls before cooking.

To ensure that meat is properly cooked, an HHA should use a meat thermometer to verify that the food has reached a safe temperature. Metal thermometers and other metal objects should not be placed in microwave ovens.

Frying: Frying uses a lot of fat and is the least healthy way to cook. HHAs should avoid frying foods for clients.

Fresh, uncooked foods: Many fruits and vegetables have the most nutrients when eaten fresh, as in salads (Fig. 6-7). However, fresh fruits and vegetables may be difficult for some clients to chew or digest. Fruits and vegetables should be washed well to remove any chemicals or pesticides.

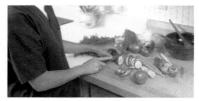

Fig. 6-7. Many fruits and vegetables have the most nutrients when eaten uncooked and fresh.

Preparing Mechanically Altered Diets

For soft, mechanical soft, or pureed diets, foods are prepared with blenders, food processors, meat grinders, or cutting utensils. Chopped foods are foods that have been cut up into very small pieces. When chopping food, use a sharp knife and a clean cutting board (separate boards for raw meat and for vegetables and other foods). Grinding breaks the foods up into even smaller pieces. Pureed foods are cooked and then ground very fine or strained. A little liquid is added to give them the consistency of baby food. Grinding and pureeing can be done in a blender or food processor. However, fruits and vegetables can also be pureed by pushing them through a colander with the back of a spoon.

All equipment used must be kept very clean to help prevent infection and illness. Take the blender or food processor apart after every use. Wash each piece that has come in contact with food in hot, soapy water, and rinse thoroughly. Wash the cutting board after each use. This is especially important after chopping raw meat, poultry, and fish. Wash it with soap or in the dishwasher before using it again. Allow cutting board to air dry.

Changing the texture of food may make it lose its appeal. Season it according to the client's preferences to make it more appealing. Talk about the food being served using positive words. Pureeing also causes nutrients to be lost, so vitamin supplements may be ordered. Constipation and dehydration are complications of a pureed diet. It is very important to follow directions exactly.

Preparing Nutritional Supplements

Illness and injury may call for nutritional supplements to be added into the client's diet. Certain medications also change the need for nutrients. Nutritional supplements may come in a powdered form or liquid form. Powdered supplements need to be mixed with a liquid before being taken; the care plan will include instructions on how much liquid to add.

When preparing supplements, make sure the supplement is mixed thoroughly. Make sure the client takes it at the ordered time. Clients who are ill, tired, or in pain may not have much of an appetite. It may take a long time for them to drink a large glass of a thick liquid. Be patient and encouraging. If a client does not want to drink the supplement, do not insist that he do so. However, do report this to your supervisor.

Guidelines: Safe Food Storage

G   Buy cold food last; get it home fast. After shopping, put away refrigerated foods first.

G   Keep it safe; refrigerate. Maintain refrigerator temperature between 36° and 40°F. Maintain freezer temperature at 0°F. Do not re-freeze items after they have been thawed.

G   Use small containers that seal tightly. Foods cool more quickly when stored in smaller containers. Store with enough room around them for air circulation. Never leave foods out for more than two hours. To prevent dry foods, such as cornmeal and flour, from becoming infested with insects, store them in tightly-sealed containers. Check dry storage areas periodically for signs of insects and rodents.

G   Check the expiration dates on foods, especially perishables. Check the refrigerator frequently for spoiled foods. Discard any you find.

Composting

Clients may use scraps left over from food preparation, food that was not eaten, or expired food to make compost. Compost is a mixture of decaying food and garden waste that is used to improve and fertilize soil. Another benefit of composting is that it reduces the amount of waste sent to landfills. Only certain items can be composted. Fruits and vegetables (including rinds and cores), egg shells, coffee grounds and filters, tea bags, old bread and crackers (and other items made from flour), grains, many types of expired boxed foods, and spices can be composted. Meats, fish, dairy products, grease, and oils cannot be composted. If your client has a compost bin, follow instructions about what to compost. If in doubt about what can be put into the bin, ask your client or supervisor for help.

Assisting a client with eating

Equipment: meal, eating utensils, clothing protector if appropriate, 2-3 napkins, wipes, or washcloths

1. Wash your hands.

2. Explain the procedure to the client, speaking clearly, slowly, and directly. Maintain face-to-face contact whenever possible.

3. Raise the head of the bed or use pillows to make sure that the client is in an upright sitting position (at a 90-degree angle).

4. If bed is adjustable, adjust bed height to where you will be able to sit at the client's eye level. Lock bed wheels.

5. Help the client wash her hands with hand wipes or washcloth if client cannot do it herself.

6. Help client put on clothing protector if desired.

7. Sit facing client at the client's eye level (Fig. 6-8). Sit on the stronger side if the client has one-sided weakness.

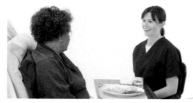

Fig. 6-8. The client should be sitting upright, and the HHA should be sitting at her eye level.

8. Tell the client what foods are on the plate. Ask client what she would like to eat first.

9. Check the temperature of the food. Test the temperature of the food by putting your hand over the dish to sense the heat. Do not touch food to test its temperature. If you think the food is too hot, do not blow on it to cool it. Offer other food to give it time to cool.

10. Using utensils, offer the food in bite-sized pieces. Tell the client the content of each bite of food offered. Alternate types of food offered, allowing for client's preferences. Do not feed all of one type before offering another type. Make sure the client's mouth is empty before the next bite or sip.

11. Offer sips of beverage to client throughout the meal. If you are holding the cup, touch it to the client's lips before you tip it. Give small, frequent sips.

12. Talk with the client during the meal. It makes mealtime more enjoyable. Do not rush the client.

13. Use washcloths, napkins, or wipes to wipe food from the client's mouth and hands as needed during the meal. Wipe mouth and hands again at the end of the meal.

14. Remove the clothing protector if used. Put it in the proper container. Remove the tray or dishes and put in proper area.

15. Assist the client to a comfortable position. Keep client in the

upright position for at least 30 minutes if ordered. Make sure bed is free from crumbs.

16. If you raised an adjustable bed, return it to its lowest position.

17. Wash your hands.

18. Document the client's intake if required and any observations. How did the client tolerate being upright for the meal? Did the client eat well? What foods did the client eat or not eat? Report any swallowing difficulties to your supervisor.

Managing Time and Money

Managing Time

HHAs must manage their time and energy efficiently. The following are guidelines to work as efficiently as possible:

Guidelines: Working Efficiently

G   Distribute tasks. Look at the client care plan and your assignments. Note the assigned housekeeping tasks. Divide the tasks and schedule them for the week and the month. Make sure all your assignments can be completed in the time you have.

G   Prioritize tasks. Prioritizing your tasks is an important time and energy management skill. Think about the jobs you want to complete throughout the day. Which ones must be done immediately? Which ones must be done at a certain time? Which activities are not absolutely essential and could be put off? Spend time on activities that are most important first.

G   Simplify tasks. Learn to simplify your tasks. Take time to think about how you will go about doing a task. Try to eliminate a few steps but still get the same result.

G   Be realistic. You may not be able to get everything done even if you plan carefully. When tasks take longer than you expected, or unexpected tasks need to be done, be realistic about what you can do. Do not be afraid to change your plan. Be flexible.

Many of the following ideas for managing time on the job can be used to manage personal time as well:

Plan ahead. Planning is the single best way to manage time better.

Prioritize. Identify the most important things to get done and do these first.

Make a schedule. Write out the hours of the day and fill in what needs to be done and when.

Combine activities. Home health aides can prepare tomorrow's dinner while the laundry is in the dryer, which combines two important tasks. Work more efficiently whenever possible.

Get help. It is a simple reality that it is not possible for an HHA to do everything, and he should not be afraid to ask for help.

Work Plan

The client care plan and the HHA's assignments will explain the tasks that are required. The HHA can develop her own work plan. This will allow her to finish all of the assigned tasks as quickly and efficiently as possible. For each day or block of time an HHA will spend in a home, she should list all the tasks she must complete and then prioritize them. The most important should be marked *1*, the next most important *2*, and so on. Finally, the HHA can write out a schedule for the day, filling in the highest priority tasks first. If there are tasks that must be done at a certain time, those tasks must be put on the schedule at the appropriate time. Tasks should be distributed so that the HHA is not trying to do all the house cleaning in one afternoon. She may then end up with no time to bathe or care for a client. Simplifying tasks whenever possible will allow the HHA to accomplish more.

Following an established work plan means more can be done in less time. It will also allow clients and families to know what to expect. The HHA may even want to discuss the plan with a client or family member as she is making it up or when it is finished. Some people appreciate knowing what will be happening in their homes at any given time.

Occasionally, an HHA may be asked to do something that is not in the care plan or her assignments. Several things can help an HHA handle requests that she must refuse. First, she must explain that she is only allowed to do tasks assigned in the care plan. She can explain that nurses familiar with the client's condition give her assignments. It is helpful for the HHA to emphasize that she would like to help, but that she is limited to the tasks outlined in the care plan and her assignments. After explaining this to the client, she should contact her supervisor and discuss the request. The supervisor may add the task requested by the client to the HHA's assignments. It is possible it was left out by mistake. The HHA should document the client's request and the actions she took to address it.

Client's Money

Different states and employers have different regulations and policies regarding healthcare employees handling clients' money. An HHA must find out from his employer whether he will be expected to handle clients' money. If he is not allowed to handle money, he should never agree to do so, even occasionally. He could get himself and his employer into serious trouble.

Guidelines: Handling a Client's Money

G   Never use a client's money for your own needs, even if you plan to pay it back. This is considered stealing. You could lose your job and/ or be arrested.

G   Estimate the amount of money you will need before requesting it. You may need to take things off your list or estimate the total bill as you go along in the store to stay within the money allotted.

G   Take checks, rather than cash, when possible. Have the client or family member fill out the name of the store. A signed check that is not made out is as good as cash.

G   Get a receipt for every purchase. This proves how much you spent and gives a record for you and the client.

G   Return receipts and change to client or family member immediately. Do not wait until the end of the day or week to settle up. Do it right away while everything is fresh in your mind.

G   Keep a record of money you have spent. Follow your agency's policies for documenting money transactions. Write down how much you spent and where. Note any change returned to client. The better record you have, the smaller the chance of misunderstanding.

G   Keep a client's cash separate from yours. If you must use the client's cash, do not put it in your own wallet. Keep it in a separate, safe place. Do the same with change. This will prevent confusion.

G   Never offer money advice to a client. You should not even refer a client to others regarding their financial matters.

G   Your clients' financial matters are confidential. Never discuss your clients' money matters with anyone.

VII. Caring For Yourself

The first six sections of this book introduce readers to the home health care setting. They cover the knowledge, skills, and qualities a person needs to work as a home health aide. This final section is more personal. It addresses the reader directly. This chapter includes information on education and career, as well as how to manage stress and stay healthy.

Continuing Education

Each state has different requirements for maintaining certification. Be familiar with the requirements. Follow them exactly or you will not be able to keep working. Ask your instructor or employer for the requirements in your state. You may also be able to check online with your state's department of health, education, or another state agency. You should know how many hours of in-service education are required per year. You also need to know how long an absence from working is allowed without retraining or recertification.

Some states have a registry for home health aides (HHAs) like the ones they maintain for certified nursing assistants (CNAs). Certified nursing assistants who are included in the state registry need to work a certain number of hours in a long-term care facility to remain in the registry. Home health aides may have similar requirements. Ask your employer how best to maintain your certification.

The federal government requires that home health aides have a 12-hour minimum of continuing education each year. Many states require more. In-service continuing education courses help you keep your knowledge and skills fresh. Classes also provide more information about certain medical conditions, challenges in working with clients, or regulation changes. You need to be up-to-date on the latest that is expected of you.

Your employer may be responsible for offering in-service courses. However, you are responsible for attending and completing them. You must do the following:

- Sign up for the course or find out where it is offered.
- Attend all class sessions.
- Pay attention and complete all the class requirements.
- Make the most of your in-service programs. Participate during class.
- Keep original copies of all certificates and records of your successful attendance so you can prove you took the class.

Stress Management

Stress is the state of being frightened, excited, confused, in danger, or irritated. It is often thought that only bad things cause stress. However, positive situations cause stress, too. For example, getting married or having a baby are usually positive situations. But both can bring enormous stress because of the changes they bring to a person's life.

You may be thrilled when you get a new job as a home health aide. But starting work may also cause you stress. You may be afraid of making mistakes, excited about earning money or helping people, or confused about your new duties. Learning how to recognize stress and what causes it is helpful. Then you can master a few simple techniques for relaxing and learn to manage stress.

A stressor is something that causes stress. Anything can be a stressor. Some examples include the following:

- Divorce
- Marriage
- New baby
- Parenthood
- Children growing up
- Children leaving home
- Feeling unprepared for a task
- Starting a new job
- Problems at work
- New responsibilities at work
- Feeling unsupported at work (not enough guidance and resources)
- Losing a job
- Supervisors
- Coworkers
- Clients
- Illness
- Finances

Stress is not only an emotional response. It is also a physical response. When a person experiences stress, changes occur in the body. The endocrine system produces more of the hormone adrenaline. This can increase nervous system response, heart rate, respiratory rate, and blood pressure. This is why, in stressful situations, your heart beats fast, you breathe hard, and you may feel warm or perspire.

Each person has a different tolerance level for stress. What one person would find overwhelming might not bother another person. A person's tolerance for stress depends on personality, life experiences, and physical health.

Guidelines: Managing Stress

To manage stress in your life, develop healthy dietary, exercise, and lifestyle habits:

G   Eat nutritious foods.

G   Exercise regularly. You can exercise alone or with a partner (Fig. 7-1).

G   Get enough sleep.

G   Drink only in moderation.

G   Do not smoke.

G   Find time at least a few times a week to do something relaxing.

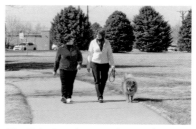

Fig. 7-1. Regular exercise, such as walking, is one healthy way to decrease stress.

Not managing stress can cause many problems. Some of these problems will affect how well you do your job. Signs that you are not managing stress include the following:

- Showing anger or being abusive to clients
- Arguing with your supervisor about assignments
- Having poor relationships with coworkers and clients
- Complaining about your job and your responsibilities
- Feeling work-related burnout (burnout is a state of mental or physical exhaustion caused by stress)
- Feeling tired even when you are rested
- Having trouble focusing on clients and procedures

Stress can seem overwhelming when you try to handle it by yourself. Often just talking about stress can help you manage it better. Sometimes another person can offer helpful suggestions. You may think of new ways to handle stress just by talking it through with another person. Get help from one or more of these resources when managing stress:

- Your supervisor or another member of the care team for work-related stress (Fig. 7-2)
- Your family
- Your friends
- A support group
- Your place of worship
- Your doctor
- A local mental health agency
- Any phone hotline that deals with related problems (check the Internet)

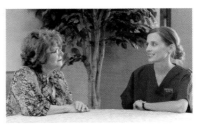

Fig. 7-2. *A supervisor is an appropriate resource for an HHA to talk to regarding stress.*

It is not appropriate to talk to your clients or their family members about your personal or job-related stress.

Developing a plan to manage stress can be helpful. The plan can include nice things you will do for yourself every day and things to do in stressful situations. Before making a plan, you first need to answer these questions:

- What are the sources of stress in my life?
- When do I most often feel stress?
- What effects of stress do I see in my life?
- What can I change to decrease the stress I feel?
- What do I have to learn to cope with because I cannot change it?

When you have answered these questions, you will have a clearer picture of the challenges you face. Then you can try to come up with strategies for managing stress.

Your Career

Specialty training for HHAs is additional training to prepare an aide to care for clients with specific medical conditions. When a person becomes specialized, he or she learns as much as possible about that type of care in order to develop more advanced skills than those taught in basic training programs. The specialty-trained HHA has more education and more experience than other aides. He or she will be a better prepared caregiver. If you are interested in specialty training, consider the following:

- Choose a specialty that you seem to be more interested in than any other. Doing what you like to do every day is very important.

- Choose a specialty that your agency has the most referrals for, or that you know you can put to use in your particular area.

- Choose a program that is well-written and designed especially for your level of education and skills.

- Read as much as you can about the condition you are specializing in on your own.

- Discuss being assigned these types of clients with your supervisor.

- Talk to your clients who have this medical condition to gain some insight into their lives. Find out how they are affected from day to day.

After you are hired at an agency, there may be times you will need to make a complaint or voice a concern about some part of your job. Do not be afraid to do this, but do it carefully.

Think about the problem. Some major problems must be reported right away. For example, if a client, family member, or coworker threatens you, report this to your supervisor immediately. Other problems may work themselves out in time. If a new client seems rude, it is possible that he or she feels uncomfortable with new people or does not understand your role. You may want to wait several days or weeks to see if things improve before making a complaint. Know which problems should be reported immediately to your supervisor.

Plan what you will say. Think through and even write out what you will say to your supervisor. This will help you present your complaint clearly and completely.

Do not get emotional. Some situations may be very upsetting. However, you will be more effective in communicating and problem-solving if you can keep your emotions out of it. Share your feelings about a situation—whether you are mad, hurt, or annoyed—with a friend (while maintaining confidentiality). Tell your supervisor the facts.

Do not hesitate to communicate situations that you feel are important or that may put you or a client at risk. One common problem in home care is aides not reporting when they feel unsafe at a particular client's home. In this case, not complaining can prove dangerous for you and the client. Always report to your supervisor any situation in which you feel you or the client is at risk of harm, even if the situation involves the client's family or friends.

If you decide to change jobs, be responsible. Always give your employer at least two weeks' written notice that you will be leaving. Otherwise, assignments may be left uncovered, or other aides may have to work more until the agency fills your spot. In addition, future employers may talk with past supervisors. People who change jobs too often or who do not give notice before leaving are less likely to be hired.

Look back over all you have learned in this program. Your work as a home health aide is very important. Every day may be different and challenging. In a hundred ways every week you will offer help that only a caring person like you can provide.

Do not forget to value the work you have chosen to do. It is important. For your clients, your work can mean the difference between living at home and living in a care facility. It can mean living with independence and dignity versus living without. The difference you make is sometimes life versus death. Look in the face of each of your clients and know that you are doing important work. Look in a mirror when you get home and be proud of how you make your living.

Being able to reflect on how you spend your time is an important life skill. Learn ways to fully appreciate that what you do has great meaning. Few jobs have the challenges and rewards of home health care. Congratulate yourself for choosing a path that includes helping others along the way.

Abbreviations

$\bar{a}$	before
ABR	absolute bedrest
ac, a.c.	before meals
ADLs	activities of daily living
AIDS	acquired immune deficiency syndrome
am, AM	morning, before noon
amb	ambulate, ambulatory
amt	amount
ap	apical
as tol	as tolerated
ax.	axillary (armpit)
BID, b.i.d	two times a day
BM	bowel movement
BP, B/P	blood pressure
BPM	beats per minute
BRP	bathroom privileges
$\bar{c}$	with
C	Centigrade
cath.	catheter
CBC	complete blood count
CBR	complete bedrest
C. diff	*clostridium difficile*
CHF	congestive heart failure
c/o	complains of
COPD	chronic obstructive pulmonary disease
CPR	cardiopulmonary resuscitation
CVA	cerebrovascular accident, stroke
DNR	do not resuscitate
DOB	date of birth
DON	director of nursing
Dx, dx	diagnosis
EMS	emergency medical services
F	Fahrenheit
FF	force fluids
ft	foot
F/U, f/u	follow-up
FWB	full weight-bearing
h, hr, hr.	hour
H_2O	water
H/A, HA	headache
HBV	hepatitis B virus
HHA	home health aide
HIPAA	Health Insurance Portability and Accountability Act
HIV	human immunodeficiency virus
HOB	head of bed
ht	height
HTN	hypertension
hyper	above normal, too fast, rapid
hypo	low, less than normal
I&O	intake and output

inc	incontinent	q̄	every
isol	isolation	q2h	every two hours
IV, I.V.	intravenous (within a vein)	q3h	every three hours
		q4h	every four hours
lab	laboratory	R	respirations, rectal
lb.	pound	rehab	rehabilitation
LTC	long-term care	RF	restrict fluids
meds	medications	R.I.C.E.	rest, ice, compression, elevation
mL	milliliter		
mmHg	millimeters of mercury	RN	registered nurse
		R/O	rule out
MRSA	methicillin-resistant *Staphylococcus aureus*	ROM	range of motion
		s̄	without
N/A	not applicable	S&S, S/S	signs and symptoms
NKA	no known allergies	SOB	shortness of breath
NPO	nothing by mouth	spec.	specimen
NVD	nausea, vomiting, and diarrhea	stat	immediately
		std. prec.	Standard Precautions
NWB	non-weight-bearing	T., temp	temperature
O_2	oxygen	TB	tuberculosis
OOB	out of bed	TID, t.i.d.	three times a day
oz	ounce	TPR	temperature, pulse, and respiration
p̄	after		
peri care	perineal care	UTI	urinary tract infection
per os, PO	by mouth	VS, vs	vital signs
PPE	personal protective equipment	w/c, W/C	wheelchair
		wt.	weight
p.r.n., prn	when necessary		
PVD	peripheral vascular disease		
PWB	partial weight-bearing		

Glossary

abuse: purposeful mistreatment that causes physical, mental, or emotional pain or injury to someone.

acquired immune deficiency syndrome (AIDS): the final stage of HIV infection, in which infections, tumors, and central nervous system symptoms appear due to a weakened immune system that is unable to fight infection.

active neglect: the purposeful failure to provide needed care, resulting in harm to a person.

activities of daily living (ADLs): daily personal care tasks such as bathing; caring for skin, nails, hair, and teeth; dressing; toileting; eating and drinking; walking; and transferring.

advance directives: legal documents that allow people to choose what medical care they wish to have if they are unable to make those decisions themselves.

age-related macular degeneration (AMD): a condition in which the macula deteriorates, causing vision loss.

agitation: being excited, restless, or troubled.

Alzheimer's disease (AD): a progressive, incurable disease that causes tangled nerve fibers and protein deposits to form in the brain, eventually causing dementia.

ambulation: walking.

ambulatory: capable of walking.

angina pectoris: chest pain, pressure, or discomfort.

anorexia: an eating disorder in which a person does not eat or exercises excessively to lose weight.

antimicrobial: an agent that destroys, resists, or prevents the development of pathogens.

anxiety: uneasiness or fear, often about a situation or condition.

arthritis: a general term that refers to inflammation of the joints that causes stiffness, pain, and decreased mobility.

aspiration: the inhalation of food, fluid, or foreign material into the lungs.

asthma: a chronic inflammatory disease that causes difficulty with breathing, coughing and wheezing.

atrophy: the wasting away, decreasing in size, and weakening of muscles from lack of use.

bipolar disorder: a type of depression that causes a person to swing from periods of deep depression to periods of extreme activity; also called manic-depressive illness.

bloodborne pathogens: microorganisms found in human blood, body fluids, draining wounds, and mucous membranes that can cause infection and disease in humans.

body mechanics: the way the parts of the body work together when a person moves.

bronchitis: an irritation and inflammation of the lining of the bronchi.

cardiopulmonary resuscitation (CPR): medical procedures used when a person's heart or lungs have stopped working.

catheter: a thin tube inserted into the body to drain or inject fluids.

cerebrovascular accident (CVA): a condition that occurs when blood supply to a part of the brain is blocked or a blood vessel leaks or ruptures within the brain; also called stroke.

chain of command: the line of authority within an agency.

chronic: long-term or long-lasting.

chronic obstructive pulmonary disorder (COPD): a chronic, incurable lung disease that causes difficulty breathing.

cognitive: related to thinking and learning.

colostomy: surgically-created opening through the abdomen into the large intestine to allow feces to be expelled.

combative: violent or hostile behavior.

combustion: the process of burning.

compassionate: being caring, concerned, considerate, empathetic, and understanding.

confidentiality: the legal and ethical principle of keeping information private.

congestive heart failure (CHF): a condition in which the heart is no longer able to pump effectively; blood backs up into the heart instead of circulating.

conscientious: guided by a sense of right and wrong; principled.

constipation: the inability to eliminate stool, or the infrequent, difficult, and often painful elimination of a hard, dry stool.

constrict: to narrow.

contracture: the permanent and often painful shortening of a muscle or tendon, usually due to lack of activity.

culture: a system of learned behaviors, practiced by a group of people, that is considered to be the tradition of that people and is passed on from one generation to the next.

cyanotic: skin that is blue or gray.

dangle: to sit up with the legs hanging over the side of the bed in order to regain balance and stabilize blood pressure.

dehydration: a serious condition that results from inadequate fluid in the body.

dementia: the serious loss of mental abilities, such as thinking, remembering, reasoning, and communicating.

diabetes: a condition in which the pancreas produces too little insulin or does not properly use insulin.

diabetic ketoacidosis (DKA): a complication of diabetes that is caused by having too little insulin; also called hyperglycemia.

diarrhea: frequent elimination of liquid or semi-liquid feces.

diastolic: second measurement of blood pressure; phase when the heart relaxes or rests.

digestion: the process of preparing food physically and chemically so that it can be absorbed into the cells.

dilate: to widen.

direct contact: a way of transmitting pathogens through touching the infected person or his or her secretions.

disorientation: confusion about person, place, or time.

draw sheet: an extra sheet placed on top of a bottom sheet; used for moving clients in bed.

dysphagia: difficulty swallowing.

dyspnea: difficulty breathing.

elimination: the process of expelling solid wastes (made up of the waste products of food) that are not absorbed into the cells.

emesis: the act of vomiting, or ejecting stomach contents through the mouth and/or nose.

emotional lability: laughing or crying without any reason or when it is inappropriate.

empathetic: being able to identify with the feelings of others.

epilepsy: an illness of the brain that produces seizures.

ethics: the knowledge of right and wrong.

exposure control plan: plan designed to eliminate or reduce employee exposure to infectious material.

expressive aphasia: trouble communicating thoughts through speech or writing.

first aid: emergency care given immediately to an injured person.

flammable: easily ignited and capable of burning quickly.

fluid balance: taking in and eliminating equal amounts of fluid.

foot drop: a weakness of muscles in the feet and ankles that causes problems with the ability to flex the ankles and walk normally.

fracture: a broken bone.

gait belt: a belt made of canvas or other heavy material used to help people who are who are weak, unsteady, or uncoordinated to stand, sit, or walk; also called a transfer belt.

gastroesophageal reflux disease (GERD): a chronic condition in which the liquid contents of the stomach back up into the esophagus.

glands: organs that produce and secrete chemicals called hormones.

glaucoma: a condition in which the fluid inside the eyeball is unable to drain; increased pressure inside the eye causes damage that often leads to blindness.

hand hygiene: washing hands with either plain or antiseptic soap and water and using alcohol-based hand rubs.

Health Insurance Portability and Accountability Act (HIPAA): a federal law that requires health information be kept private and secure and that organizations take special steps to protect this information.

health maintenance organizations (HMOs): a method of health insurance in which a person has to use a particular doctor or group of doctors except in case of emergency.

hemiparesis: weakness on one side of the body.

hemiplegia: paralysis on one side of the body.

hepatitis: inflammation of the liver caused by certain viruses and other factors, such as alcohol abuse, some medications, and trauma.

homeostasis: the condition in which all of the body's systems are working at their best.

hormones: chemical substances created by the body that control numerous body functions.

human immunodeficiency virus (HIV): virus that attacks the body's immune system and gradually disables it; eventually can cause AIDS.

hygiene: practices to keep bodies clean and healthy.

hypertension (HTN): high blood pressure, measuring 140/90 or higher.

incident report: a report that must be completed when an accident, problem, or other unexpected event occurs during a visit.

incontinence: the inability to control the bladder or bowels.

indirect contact: a way of transmitting pathogens by touching something contaminated by the infected person.

infection prevention: the set of methods practiced in healthcare facilities and other settings to prevent and control the spread of disease.

infectious: contagious.

insulin reaction: complication of diabetes that can result from either too much insulin or too little food; also known as hypoglycemia.

intake: the fluid a person consumes; also called input.

intravenous (IV): into a vein.

intravenous therapy (IV therapy): the delivery of medication, nutrition, or fluids through a person's vein.

laws: rules set by the government to help people live peacefully together and to ensure order and safety.

liability: a legal term that means someone can be held responsible for harming someone else.

major depressive disorder: a type of depression that causes withdrawal, lack of energy, and loss of interest in activities, as well as other symptoms; also called major depression.

Medicaid: a medical assistance program for people with low incomes, as well as for people with disabilities.

medical asepsis: refers to practices such as handwashing that reduce, remove, and control the spread of microorganisms.

Medicare: a federal health insurance program for people who are 65 or older, are disabled, or are ill and cannot work.

metabolism: physical and chemical processes by which substances are produced or broken down into energy or products for use by the body.

microorganism (MO): a living thing or organism that is so small that it can be seen only under a microscope; also called a microbe.

mucous membranes: the membranes that line body cavities that open to the outside of the body, such as the linings of the mouth, nose, eyes, rectum, or genitals.

multiple sclerosis (MS): a progressive disease in which the myelin sheath covering nerves breaks down over time; without this protective covering, nerves cannot conduct impulses to and from the brain in a normal way.

myocardial infarction (MI): a condition that occurs when the heart muscle does not receive enough oxygen because blood vessels are blocked; also called heart attack.

neglect: the failure to provide needed care that results in physical, mental, or emotional harm to a person.

negligence: actions, or the failure to act or provide the proper care, that result in unintended injury to a person.

neuropathy: numbness, tingling, and pain in the feet and legs.

nonverbal communication: communicating without using words.

Occupational Safety and Health Administration (OSHA): a federal government agency that makes rules to protect workers from hazards on the job.

orthotic device: a device that helps support and align a limb and improve its functioning; also called orthosis.

osteoporosis: a disease that causes bones to become porous and brittle, causing them to break easily.

ostomy: a surgically-created opening from an area inside the body to the outside.

output: all fluid that is eliminated from the body; includes fluid in urine, feces, vomitus, perspiration, moisture that is exhaled in the air, and wound drainage.

oxygen therapy: the administration of oxygen to increase the supply of oxygen to the lungs.

palliative care: care that focuses on pain relief, comfort, and dignity for a person who is very sick and/or dying.

passive neglect: the unintentional failure to provide needed care, resulting in physical, mental, or emotional harm to a person.

pathogen: microorganism that is capable of causing infection and disease.

perineal care: care of the genital and anal area.

perseveration: the repetition of words, phrases, questions, or actions.

personal protective equipment (PPE): equipment that helps protect employees from serious workplace injuries or illnesses resulting from contact with workplace hazards.

phobia: an intense form of anxiety or fear.

physical abuse: any treatment, intentional or not, that causes harm to a person's body.

policy: a course of action that should be taken every time a certain situation occurs.

preferred provider organizations (PPOs): a network of providers that contract to provide health services to a group of people.

pressure ulcer: a serious wound resulting from skin breakdown; also called decubitus ulcer, pressure sore, or bed sore.

procedure: a method, or way, of doing something.

prosthesis: a device that replaces a body part that is missing or deformed because of an accident, injury, illness, or birth defect; used to improve a person's ability to function and/or his appearance.

psychological abuse: emotional harm caused by threatening, scaring, humiliating, intimidating, isolating, or insulting a person, or by treating him as a child; also includes verbal abuse.

psychosocial needs: needs that involve social interaction, emotions, intellect, and spirituality.

range of motion (ROM): exercises that put a joint through its full arc of motion.

receptive aphasia: difficulty understanding spoken or written words.

respiration: the process of breathing air into the lungs and exhaling air out of the lungs.

scabies: contagious skin infection caused by a tiny mite burrowing into the skin, where it lays eggs; causes intense itching and a skin rash that may look like thin burrow tracks.

schizophrenia: a form of mental illness that affects a person's ability to think, communicate, make decisions, and understand reality.

scope of practice: defines the tasks that healthcare providers are legally allowed to do and how to do them correctly.

sexual abuse: the forcing of a person to perform or participate in sexual acts against his or her will; includes unwanted touching, exposing oneself, and the sharing of pornographic material.

sexually transmitted infections (STIs): infections caused by sexual contact with infected people; signs and symptoms are not always apparent.

sharps: needles or other sharp objects.

shearing: rubbing or friction that results from the skin moving one way and the bone underneath it remaining fixed or moving in the opposite direction.

shingles: non-contagious skin rash caused by the varicella-zoster virus (VZV), which is the same virus that causes chickenpox; causes pain, tingling, itching, and a rash of fluid-filled blisters.

specimen: a sample that is used for analysis in order to try to make a diagnosis.

sputum: thick mucus coughed up from the lungs.

Standard Precautions: a method of infection prevention in which all blood, body fluids, non-intact skin, and mucous membranes are treated as if they were infected with an infectious disease.

stoma: an artificial opening in the body.

sundowning: becoming restless and agitated in the late afternoon, evening, or night.

systolic: first measurement of blood pressure; phase when the heart is at work, contracting and pushing the blood from the left ventricle of the heart.

tactful: showing sensitivity and having a sense of what is appropriate when dealing with others.

terminal illness: a disease or condition that will eventually cause death.

transfer belt: a belt made of canvas or other heavy material that is used to help people who are weak, unsteady, or uncoordinated to stand, sit, or walk; also called gait belt.

tuberculosis (TB): a highly contagious lung disease caused by a bacterium that is carried on mucous droplets suspended in the air.

tumor: a cluster of abnormally-growing cells.

validating: giving value to or approving.

verbal abuse: the use of spoken or written words, pictures, or gestures that threaten, embarrass, or insult a person.

Index

Important Names/Numbers

Abuse Hotline

Alzheimer's Association (local)

Area Agency on Aging

Church/Spiritual Advisor

Dietitian

Errand Service

Family Members

Fire Department

HHA Agency

Hospice

Meals on Wheels

Medical Supply Company

Natural Disaster Information Line

Pharmacist

Physician

Poison Control Center

Police Department (Non-Emergency)

Public Transportation

Senior Citizens' Center

Supervisor

Transportation Services

Other Resources:

Community Resources

Here are a few of the many community resources available to help clients meet different needs:

- Eldercare Locator, a public service of the U.S. Administration on Aging (eldercare.gov or 800-677-1116)

- The National Resource Center on LGBT Aging (lgbtagingcenter.org or 212-741-2247)

- Alzheimer's Association (alz.org or 800-272-3900)

- American Cancer Society (cancer.org or 800-227-2345)

- AIDSinfo, a service of the U.S. Department of Health and Human Services (aidsinfo.nih.gov or 800-448-0440)

- Meals on Wheels Association of America (MOWAA) (mowaa.org or 888-998-6325)

- American Association on Intellectual and Developmental Disabilities (AAIDD) (aaidd.org or 202-387-1968)

- The National Institute of Mental Health (NIMH) (nimh.nih.gov or 866-615-6464)

- The National Hospice and Palliative Care Organization (NHPCO) (nhpco.org or 800-658-8898)